SpringerBriefs in Public Health

SpringerBriefs in Public Health present concise summaries of cutting-edge research and practical applications from across the entire field of public health, with contributions from medicine, bioethics, health economics, public policy, biostatistics, and sociology.

The focus of the series is to highlight current topics in public health of interest to a global audience, including health care policy; social determinants of health; health issues in developing countries; new research methods; chronic and infectious disease epidemics; and innovative health interventions.

Featuring compact volumes of 50 to 125 pages, the series covers a range of content from professional to academic. Possible volumes in the series may consist of timely reports of state-of-the art analytical techniques, reports from the field, snapshots of hot and/or emerging topics, elaborated theses, literature reviews, and in-depth case studies. Both solicited and unsolicited manuscripts are considered for publication in this series.

Briefs are published as part of Springer's eBook collection, with millions of users worldwide. In addition, Briefs are available for individual print and electronic purchase.

Briefs are characterized by fast, global electronic dissemination, standard publishing contracts, easy-to-use manuscript preparation and formatting guidelines, and expedited production schedules. We aim for publication 8–12 weeks after acceptance.

More information about this series at http://www.springer.com/series/10138

Prem Misir

COVID-19 and Health System Segregation in the US

Racial Health Disparities and Systemic Racism

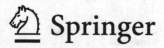 Springer

Prem Misir
School of Public Health
The University of the South Pacific, Solomon Islands (Immediate Past)
Honiara, Solomon Islands

ISSN 2192-3698   ISSN 2192-3701   (electronic)
SpringerBriefs in Public Health
ISBN 978-3-030-88765-0   ISBN 978-3-030-88766-7   (eBook)
https://doi.org/10.1007/978-3-030-88766-7

This Springer imprint is published by the registered company Springer Nature Switzerland AG
The registered company address is: Gewerbestrasse 11, 6330 Cham, Switzerland

Foreword

Human beings have a strong need for perspective. How, for example, does one make sense of all of the events that swirl about us, particularly in the face of a pandemic? COVID-19 has, since its inception, transformed our understanding of life, death, and health. The pandemic's impact on the world's economy as well as on the political structures of the world's governments has been so enormous that one struggles to develop the language to describe it. How do we achieve some perspective, some method for making sense of all that has happened in our struggles with the virus? How can that perspective arm us for the future?

Perhaps we can begin with a simple but challenging question: How will future historians view this period of history? If we could make use of the historian's 20/20 hindsight, what would we discover in examining the short-term and long-term impacts of the pandemic on life in the USA? We would clearly see, perhaps more than we are able to see right now, the fruits of racism and marginalization as a fundamental element of US history and as a driving factor in the high rates of COVID-19 hospitalizations and mortality among Black and Brown communities in the USA.

In this book, Dr. Prem Misir examines the pandemic in the USA and its devastation through the prism of racism. The high rates of COVID-19 infection in communities of color in this nation are a direct consequence, he shows, of the systemic exploitation of those communities. Moreover, the history of that exploitation began more than 400 years ago. As he points out, "Racial health disparities and segregated health care are not new to America, as differential health outcomes between Blacks and Whites were birthed at the time of the settlement at Jamestown in 1619."

The history of slavery in the USA is poorly understood by the average American, but the legacy of that era endures. It endures in the racially segregated communities that are so much a part of this nation's urban growth and development and it endures, as shall be shown, in the devastation of COVID-19. Pandemics exploit marginal communities and their social and economic disadvantage. Public health policies and interventions are increasingly mindful of this challenge. Much of what must be done in the face of present and future epidemics, it is argued, must be to empower those communities to rebuild and to confront the racism that has been the driving force behind racial inequalities in health.

More importantly, as the author argues, "there is no question of the overwhelming evidence of racial health disparities experienced by Blacks and other historically racially disadvantaged groups. The necessity for pursuing solutions to end systemic racism is now."

Robert E. Fullilove
Professor, Sociomedical Sciences at the
Columbia University Medical Center
Associate Dean, Community and Minority Affairs
New York, NY, USA
August 2, 2021

Preface

Shortly after my Christmas/New Year vacation in 2019/2020, I returned to the USA, only to be greeted with COVID-19. Since the prognosis on the duration of this pandemic was emphatically pointing toward a long haul, along with the expiration of my contract at The University of the South Pacific, Solomon Islands, I made a conscious decision to author a book on COVID-19 during this period. After the usual preliminary screenings and peer evaluations, Springer Nature, the publisher in New York, approved my book manuscript proposal. Not to become distracted with pursuing any new job contract at that time, I spent 2020 and a few months into 2021 fully focused on making this book proposal a reality, a book that addresses racial health disparities in the US segregated health-care system.

Without question, America has progressed profoundly in public health, medical technology, and health care, and with the incurrence of huge health expenditures. Yet, America is tarnished with a massive persisting culture of racial inequalities and inequities. Indeed, the racial health disparities are not new, as they owed their origins to the beginnings of colonial America and its racialized social systems. But America archetypally awaits an outbreak, an epidemic, a pandemic, or some other disaster, in order to place these disparities on the radar for possible resolution.

America's social structure is deeply rooted in racial segregation, birthed since the Jamestown Settlement in 1619, and more than 50 years after the Civil Rights Act, 1964, racial segregation still persists. Segregation implies the sustainability of power through the production and reproduction of domination, against an ethnically differentiated and deprived population of color, who remain trapped in the wretchedness of marginalization, characterized by structural subordination, dependence, racial oppression, and inequality. Unsurprisingly, this perpetual level of human savagery ensures that poor people of color are denied the basics – adequate housing, employment, basic medical services, and appropriate education.

For all intents and purposes, the dispossessed communities of color constitute a White-dominated colony within the political and economic context of internal colonialism in the USA. Given this political framework, this colony is a structure of social inequality with a racial hierarchy. Socioeconomic deprivation flowing from racial residential segregation and the urban ghetto has recurrently influenced the leadership within the communities of color to perceive their lived experience of racism as not only individual and interpersonal, but also institutional.

It is an understatement to say that America has a perennial and chronic health crisis afflicting the Blacks and Brown communities of color. There is no question that Blacks and other communities of color remain demographically overrepresented in COVID-19 incidence, hospitalizations, and deaths. The devastation imposed on the racially disadvantaged groups of the poor with concomitant human rights violations in itself merits dissemination to a global audience.

The US health system functions on the doctrine of "separate but equal," where the dominant White group accesses quality health care and where Blacks and the other poor experience exposure to a lesser or zero health care. Without a doubt, the USA has in place a race and class-based segregation of health care. There is the de jure health system for all, but there is the de facto health system that generates the racial segregated health care. And for the last 20 months since January 2020, COVID-19 has constantly intensified the burden of racial health disparities on the poor and vulnerable people of color.

We deemed this study as essential in light of the human tragedy wrought by the highly transmissible COVID-19, which has refined and re-exposed the vulgarities of White-imposed racism and racial oppression in consort with persisting racial health inequalities and racial health inequities on people of color. This study is part of a larger research program on systemic racism and US health care amid racial health disparities in COVID-19 incidence, hospitalizations, comorbidity, and deaths.

This book has five chapters. Chapter 1 presents the introduction to racial health disparities, race and class-based segregation of health care, and poor clinical outcomes. Chapter 2 looks at the epidemiology of COVID-19, examining the beginnings of COVID-19, distribution of COVID-19 deaths, and mismanagement of the COVID-19 pandemic. Chapter 3 examines the White racial frame, providing a historical overview, systemic racism theories, and a research proposal to explore whether COVID-19 deaths among Whites, Blacks, and Hispanics varied by urban-rural classification. Chapter 4 presents the analysis of COVID-19 deaths in 760 counties in 50 states and DC for the period January 4, 2020–April 17, 2021. Chapter 5 theorizes on the pathways to dismantle systemic racism in health care.

I am grateful and honored that Professor Robert Fullilove, Sociomedical Sciences, Columbia University Medical Center, and Associate Dean, Community and Minority Affairs, agreed to write the foreword for this book. My engagement in several discourses with Professor Joe Feagin, Ella C. McFadden, Professor and Distinguished Professor, Texas A&M University, refined my thinking on the White racial frame. My heartfelt thanks go out to: Professor Clem Sankat, President, University of Belize; Dr. Jack Maebuta, Acting Vice-Chancellor, Solomon Islands National University, and Dr. Ramesh Sharma, Associate Professor of Instructional Design, Dr. B.R. Ambedkar University Delhi, for their endorsement of this research work. I would also express my thanks to Ms. Jerlin Seles, who facilitated the data analysis. And, indeed, I must recognize Ms. Janet Kim, Senior Editor, *Springer Nature*, who was a constant source of advice and encouragement to bring this project to a successful completion.

Prem Misir
Honiara, Solomon Islands
August 11, 2021

Endorsements

"Professor Prem Misir's book explores the demographically disproportionate impact of the highly contagious COVID-19 pandemic on African Americans and other communities of color across 50 States and the District of Columbia in the US, focusing on the epidemiology of the pathogen as well as racial health disparities. This riveting book is an essential read for anyone pursuing health promotion, prolonging life, and disease prevention."

–Jack Maebuta, PhD, Acting Vice-Chancellor, Solomon Islands National University

"Socio-economically disadvantaged groups are particularly vulnerable to gaps in access as well as quality of healthcare available to them. COVID-19 has made these inequalities starker. In most societies, ethnic, religious and racial minorities have poorer outcomes than the rest of society. While the vulnerability to COVID-19 infection is equal for all, the risk of infection is also higher for these marginalized populations. Global consensus advises the use of evidence-based decisions in the face of the coronavirus pandemic. This is what Professor Prem Misir's research-oriented book intends to do. It aims by strengthening evidence for better policy and treatment approach."

–Ramesh Sharma, PhD, Associate Professor of Instructional Design, Dr. B.R. Ambedkar University Delhi

"Prem Misir has been examining and educating us for a few decades on the imbalances of the impacts of diseases on the health and wellness of the population of our plural societies in developing countries. He has especially challenged our thinking on ethnicity and socioeconomic conditions of populations with respect to their susceptibility to disease and satisfactory health care. Prem has turned his attention to COVID-19 and its impacts on the health of disadvantaged groups and on people of color within the US. This publication will inform health care administrators and medical practitioners in our own developing countries on strategies to address this dreaded disease of our lifetime."

–Clement Sankat, PhD, CEng, President, University of Belize

Contents

About the Author

Prem Misir, PhD is Former Vice-Chancellor, The University of Fiji; Former Pro Vice-Chancellor, Solomon Islands Campus and Professor and Head, School of Public Health, The University of the South Pacific. Professor Misir also was Dean, Centre for iTaukei Studies, The University of Fiji; Dean, Foundation Studies, The University of Fiji; and Dean, University–Wide Program, The University of Fiji.

Professor Misir is the holder of PhD (University of Hull, England); MPH (University of Manchester, England); MPhil (University of Surrey, England); B.S.Sc. (Honours) (Queen's University of Belfast, United Kingdom); Fellow of the Royal Society for Public Health (FRSPH, England); and Certificate, Harvard University – Improving Global Health: Focusing on Quality and Safety.

Professor Misir was Visiting Professor at the University of the West Indies; Visiting Professor, Anton de Kom University in Suriname; and Honorary Professor at the University of Central Lancashire in England. He was the former Pro-Chancellor of the University of Guyana.

In addition to journal articles, he is the author of 11 books, the most recent being: *HIV/AIDS and Adolescents: South Pacific and Caribbean*, Singapore, Palgrave Macmillan, 2019; *The Subaltern Indian Woman: Domination and Social Degradation*, Singapore, Palgrave Macmillan, 2018; and *HIV & AIDS: Knowledge and Stigma in Guyana*, University of the West Indies Press, 2013.

Chapter 1
Introduction: Segregation of Health Care

Racial Health Disparities

It is worth noting that a largely unprepared and unresponsive world was no match for the severe acute respiratory syndrome coronavirus 2 (SARS-CoV-2), the virus that causes the Coronavirus Disease 2019 (COVID-19), with 198,614,523 cases and 4,229,142 deaths worldwide on August 2, 2021 (JHU CSSE, 2021) and with an inept and unprepared US as one of the poorest performers in combating this highly contagious pathogen, running with 35,055,767 cases and 613,444 deaths on August 2, 2021 (JHU CSSE, 2021), rapidly approaching its own death rate of 675,000 in the Spanish Influenza 2018 (CDC, 2019a).

The scale of COVID-19 devastation parallels the most lethal pandemic of all time, the Spanish Flu Pandemic of 1918. Catherine Arnold (2018) referred to the Spanish Flu as the great medical holocaust, which invoked visions of the Black death of 1348, the great plague of 1665, the dreadful waves of cholera, and typhus in Europe in the 1840s. She said that with the Spanish Flu, 10 to 20% of the infected died, a third of the global population with some 50 million at that time: 17 million in India, 2% of Africa with 100,000 in Ghana, 10% of Tanzania's population, and about half a million in the USA, overall, killing more people than the Black Death. These statistics depicted the gruesome consequences and images of a pandemic that afflicted the world just over 100 years ago.

While writing about COVID-19, it is hard not to notice the pathway of this virus gaining ascendancy toward reconstructing a new world and bringing into focus a new raison d'être. This pathogen has been busy fashioning the "new normal" and, at the same time, refocusing America's attention to its racist history, racial discrimination, and White supremacy through its onslaught on the poor and vulnerable people of color, who mostly belong to the lower socioeconomic groups. The virus has refocused racial health disparities on the political radar. The Healthy People 2020 views health disparity as:

P. Misir, *COVID-19 and Health System Segregation in the US*, Springer Briefs
in Public Health, https://doi.org/10.1007/978-3-030-88766-7_1

A particular type of health difference that is closely linked with social, economic, and/or environmental disadvantage. Health disparities adversely affect groups of people who have systematically experienced greater obstacles to health based on their racial or ethnic group; religion; socioeconomic status; gender; age; mental health; cognitive, sensory, or physical disability; sexual orientation or gender identity; geographic location; or other characteristics historically linked to discrimination or exclusion (ODPHP, 2021).

Like HIV, the impact of COVID-19 on the non-White community corresponds to the overarching centuries-old racial health disparities afflicting the disadvantaged people of color. The US communities of color which are demographically overrepresented in the two concurrent pandemics, HIV and COVID-19 (Fields et al., 2021), in fact, are also battling a third pandemic, that is, systemic racism, which has been around for some 400 years and engenders a devastating perpetual public health crisis among the historically racially disadvantaged. Clearly, the policies of racial health inequities and health inequalities were formulated and implemented since 1619 at the Jamestown Settlement, where Africans were first purchased or sold as slaves.

Hence, the suggestion that racial justice and equity as national goals were abandoned subsequent to Reconstruction (Bond, 1997) is to erroneously assume that such goals were ever present in the first place. White colonists would have hardly subscribed to such national goals, especially when White-imposed racism and racial oppression were the twin pillars of the structural foundation of the original colonial and US social systems (Feagin, 2020). These twin pillars of racial injustice solidify the persisting robustness of this unswerving racist foundational reality in the present day. It may be more pertinent to perceive those national goals as racial injustice and inequity. Long before US President Joe Biden labeled the rising White supremacy as "terrorism" (NYT, 2021), there have been powerful forces at work aimed at undermining the overall Civil Rights gains, affirmative action, the social safety net, and health care for the disadvantaged, in order to mastermind a return not to the traditional overt but a covert Jim Crow environment, now fully rooted in color-blind racism. The new covert Jim Crow milieu has arrived. Thus, it is not surprising that Blacks (used interchangeably with "African Americans") remain trapped in poor health compared to non-Hispanic Whites (subsequently referred to as Whites) ever since the settlement at Jamestown in 1619.

Racial health disparities, inclusive of inequities and inequalities, remain essential power drivers of US health care, largely because of White resistance and flagrant denial of the social reality of the racially disadvantaged and marginalized poor. It took the likes of COVID-19, with its capacity as some supposed equalizer impacting all in its path, to shine the spotlight on the poor people of color, who typically experience inadequate health-care access as well as perilous exposure to the disease, due mainly to their occupancy of frontline/essential jobs. Nonetheless, at the same time, COVID-19 is on the radar exposing racial health disparities. Interestingly, COVID-19 could be the bellwether phenomenon to address the causes of these inequities (Yancy, 2020).

The continuing global untold damage of COVID-19 is following closely on the heels of the overwhelming impact of the Spanish Flu Pandemic of 1918. While the

COVID-19 pandemic has overwhelmed all the 50 States and its Territories, its impact on Blacks and the underserved populations remains direct and catastrophic. In some ways, Blacks and the underserved, that is, the marginalized, poor, and vulnerable, are constituents of the othering (De Beauvoir, 2010), making them the suspicious "others," who are perceived as inessential. Compared to the essential, that is, the dominant White group, Blacks and the marginalized poor are greatly exposed to COVID-19, as many Blacks live in poor areas with high housing density, high crime rates, and poor access to healthy foods and Blacks, as per poor crowded living conditions, are unable to engage in social distancing, an effective measure to reduce the COVID-19 infection (Yancy, 2020).

This "public health" victimization of Blacks should not be surprising, as they have been at the receiving end of poor health compared to White Americans for as long as there has been an America (Byrd & Clayton, 2012). Byrd and Clayton (2012) chronicled Blacks being the victims of the most oppressive race-based health history, noting that the Malone-Heckler report in the 1980s helped to channel the Black health crisis to the mainstream health system's consciousness. The report of the Secretary of the US Department of Health and Human Services Margaret Heckler titled *Health, United States, 1983,* submitted to Congress noted that US public health had improved significantly, where Americans had a higher life expectancy and low infant mortality and that American health displayed total improvement. But the Secretary also communicated a sad fact, possibly documented for the first time, that there was a persistent disparity in the burden of death and illness suffered by Blacks and other minority Americans compared with the US population en bloc (USDHHS, 1985–1986). These disparities are not new, as they have persisted between Blacks and Whites in the USA from the time the first settlers arrived. However, even 36 years after the 1985 Heckler Report, disparities in the life expectancy and the leading causes of death for Blacks compared with Whites were huge (Cunningham et al., 2017). This trend in increased racial health disparities is persisting, as evidenced by the disproportionate COVID-19 impact on Blacks and other people of color.

Some three decades after the Heckler report, COVID-19 arrived in the USA, and as usual with previous disease outbreaks or pandemics, it brought the growing racial health inequalities and health inequities to the surface again. In an interview with the British Medical Journal, Director of the National Institute of Allergy and Infectious Diseases (NIAID), Dr. Anthony Fauci, when asked whether this was the appropriate time to address racial health disparities in the USA, responded (Godlee & Silberner, 2020 pp. 2–3), thus:

Yes, it is a very unfortunate situation for all of these groups, not only with covid-19 but with other diseases. Look, for example, at the population of African-Americans: they're about 13% of the US population, but well over 40-45% of all new covid-19 cases are among African-Americans. They get hit by two disparities: jobs that do not allow them to easily protect themselves from the close, person-to-person contact that we know transmits the virus, and a disparately larger percentage of the underlying conditions that lead to a serious outcome—diabetes, hypertension, cardiovascular disease, obesity. There's something that we can immediately do, and that's to focus and concentrate resources and accessibility in areas that are demographically over-represented by African-Americans. If there's ever a silver lining in this, it may be that it jolts us into realizing that we have to correct disparities in minority health—because otherwise, in the next situation that we have like this, we're going to see the same painful disparity that we're seeing now.

Segregated Health System

Since the beginnings of colonial America, the USA has had a de jure segregated health care, that is, a legal segregated health system, alongside an insidious and growing Black health crisis, powered by the White racial frame, racialized social systems and a racial hierarchy. This legal segregated health system functioned within the doctrine of "separate but equal," whereby the dominant White group had access to quality health care and the people of color had to contend with a lesser or zero health care. However, the Civil Rights Act, 1964, and the Social Security Act Amendments, 1965, widely known as the Medicare bill, outlawed segregation within the health system. So by law, you would think that the USA now has a deseg-regated healthcare system. But not so fast, as the segregated health system has endured. The de jure desegregated health system exists for all by law, but it is the de facto segregated health system that is in effect: one for the White dominant group and one for the people of color, where "separation" implies and enforces inferiority in health care. The prevailing de facto and covert segregated health system, grounded in color-blind racism alongside residential segregation of huge cross-sections of the Black population, has become the new reality for people of color.

Residential segregation impacts the shape and quality of the health system vis-à-vis its link to non-primary care facilities in a disadvantaged environment, ultimately depriving Blacks of appropriate and equal access to primary care sites as a usual source of care. It means, historically, Blacks have had to utilize non-primary care sites as the emergency department (ED) and hospital outpatient departments with greater frequency than Whites (USCB, 2012), limiting the possibility to gain from primary care exposure. However, they have been utilizing the private physicians' offices (primary care site) at merely two-thirds the rate of Whites (USNCHS, 2012). Blacks' utilization of non-primary care sites as their usual source of care was also linked to poor health outcomes for several diseases (Gaskin et al., 2007). Factors that contributed to race and class-based segregation of health care disadvantaging vastly segregated Black communities are the clustering poverty and uninsured status arising from socioeconomic deprivation (male joblessness, teenage motherhood, and single parenthood) that produced the underclass. Furthermore, physicians were less likely to participate in Medicaid areas where the poor were non-White and where there was residential segregation (Gaskin et al., 2012b). By 1990, a powerful interface between residential segregation and income inequality developed to spatially segregate the poor, fully reinforced by fragile links between residential segregation, poor education, growing class segregation, and declining average incomes (Massey & Fong, 1990; Massey et al., 1991; Greene et al., 2006; Massey & Fischer, 2000).

Segregated health care was also related to geography. Gaskin et al. (2012c) studied the relationship between residential segregation and geographic access to primary care physicians in the metropolitan statistical areas (MSAs) and found that the probabilities of being a primary care physician shortage area were 67% greater for majority Black zip codes, but 27% lesser for majority Hispanic zip codes. As the amount of segregation proliferated, the probabilities of being a primary care physician shortage in the area increased for majority African American zip codes, but not for majority Hispanic and Asian zip codes. Another study (Gaskin et al., 2012a) showed that the disparities in health-care utilization were associated with both the individual's racial and ethnic identity and the racial and ethnic composition of their communities. It shows that the interventions to progress access to health-care services and to jettison health-care disparities for Blacks and Hispanics should not only concentrate on individual-level aspects but also take account of community-level factors. Kirby and Kaneda (2005) concluded that living in disadvantaged neighborhoods lessened the probability of access to a usual source of care and preventive services. It shows that a strong relationship prevailed between neighborhood disadvantage and access to health care. The studies presented in this section inferred the existential presence of de facto segregated health care, one kind that caters to the advantaged and the other kind for the poor and underclass, promoting a sustained culture of racial health disparities and inequalities, certainly powerful ingredients for sustaining the Black health crisis.

One of the characteristics of this ever-present Black health crisis (Byrd & Clayton, 2012) is the persistent race- and class-based segregation of the health system torn between the mainstream health system and the inferior health system for Blacks and the other poor populations. A system where race- and class-based inequities and inequalities emanate from every fiber of the 402-year-old health system, and are getting worse, but are perceived as normal. Let me be clear that from a formal organizational perspective, the USA currently does not have two formal distinct health systems as it had in the past, but for all intents and purposes, the current mainstream health system still generates demographically disproportionate health outcomes, disadvantaging Blacks and the underserved populations. The end products are racial health inequality and inequity.

The National Academy of Sciences, Engineering, and Medicine (National Academies of Sciences and Medicine, 2017 p. 1) presents the following definition of health equity:

> Health equity is the state in which everyone has the opportunity to attain full health potential and no one is disadvantaged from achieving this potential because of social position or any other socially defined circumstance. Health equity and opportunity are inextricably linked. Currently in the United States, the burdens of disease and poor health and the benefits of well-being and good health are inequitably distributed. This inequitable distribution is caused by social, environmental, economic, and structural factors that shape health and are themselves distributed unequally, with pronounced differences in opportunities for health.

Extrapolating from The National Academy's definition is the view that health inequities are largely the outcome of poverty, systemic racism, and discrimination where:

The present black health crisis is a continuum. After 346 years of neglect, flawed efforts were made to admit black Americans to the "mainstream" health system. Gains were significant from 1965 to 1975; however, since then black health status has eroded...Physician leadership helped to establish the slaveocracy, create the racial inferiority myths, and build the segregated health subsystem for blacks and the poor. (Byrd & Clayton, 1992 p. 189)

The race and class-based segregation of health care, rooted in slaveocracy, Jim Crow, and the new Jim Crow, remains the pillar of racial health disparities in the US health system and health care. Systemic racism was implanted in the health-care system vis-à-vis the White racial frame, where White men formulated and implemented most health-care decisions (Feagin & Bennefield, 2014). Systemic racism, embodying the principle of separation, was already embedded into the health-care law from the early nineteenth century to the early twentieth century, where legislation ensured that Blacks did not have similar access as Whites to health care, with the provision of separate and segregated health-care facilities built in the 1800s (Matthew, 2018). This victimization of Blacks is not surprising because the health system still operates on the principle of racial segregation. How so? After the Civil War and the abolition of legal slavery, several former Confederate States enacted Jim Crow laws mandating segregated facilities for Blacks and Whites. The US Supreme Court's ruling in 1896 in the *Plessy v. Ferguson*, 163 U.S. 537, which touted the phrase "separate but equal," endorsed state racial segregation laws for public facilities (GLL, 2020a). Justice Harlan presented the sole dissent. This groundbreaking case upheld the Jim Crow laws, proclaiming the constitutionality of the "separate but equal" facilities. This judicial decision paved the way for the mushrooming of separate health-care facilities through State and local segregation ordinances.

Such laws sustained its robustness until 1954, when the US Supreme Court in *Brown v. Board of Education of Topeka*, 347 U.S. 483 (1954), ruled that States could no longer uphold or institute laws permitting separate schools for Black and White students, culminating in the beginning of the end of State-sponsored segregation in education (GLL, 2020b). This momentous case affirmed that "separate educational facilities are inherently unequal," hence terminating de jure segregation, mainly in education. Then came the Hill-Burton Act of 1946 that endorsed the modernization of hospitals and further increased the number of separate hospitals nationally. The 1954 US Supreme Court ruling applied mainly to outlawing segregation in education, and thus could not impact the Hill-Burton Act of 1946, or the "separate but equal" doctrine endorsing separate hospitals for Blacks and Whites. But if there were a focus on intersecting forms of systemic discrimination in the *Brown v. Board of Education* ruling to include sex, housing, health, etc., then perhaps, the potency of the Hill-Burton law would have been dissolved as well as the institution of separate hospitals. However, it was not until 1979, when the *Cook v. Ochsner* lawsuit

(Matthew, 2018) challenged the separate but equal exclusion clause for Black and White patients and brought amendment for the Medicaid patients.

Disparities in White-Black mortality in the USA decreased during the age of anti-poverty programs in the 1960s–1980s. In those years, health-related institutions were less segregated along with decreased racial-socioeconomic differences (Krieger et al., 2008; Roberts, 2011). Nonetheless, disparities in mortality multiplied in the 1980s, with conservatives determined to end government programs, markedly advantaging communities of color (Feagin & Bennefield, 2014). However, Title VI of the 1964 Civil Rights Act prohibits discrimination and segregation in health-related institutions: "No person in the United States shall, on the grounds of race, color, or national origin, be excluded from participation in, be denied the benefits of, or be subjected to discrimination under any program or activity receiving Federal financial assistance" (U.S.C., 1964). As it stands, Title VI of the 1964 Civil Rights Act actively protects formal access to existing health care, which, however, may be inadequate in scope as per availability of services and reachability for the poor populations. The Act, however, did not address quality health care, considering the huge evidence of persisting poor clinical outcomes experienced by Blacks and other poor populations, clearly signaling that the USA has a segregated health-care system with victimization as the end product.

This concept of racial health disparities and a segregated health care is not a new phenomenon, by virtue of its persistence between Blacks and Whites in the USA from the time the first settlers arrived. "There has never been a time in the United States without racial health disparities. Although the term 'health disparities' is of recent origin, differential health outcomes between Blacks and Whites have been part of the American landscape for 400 years" (Hammonds & Reverby, 2019 p. 1348).

Even today, the US health-care system subscribes to a de facto doctrine of "separate but equal," whereby the dominant White group has access to quality health care and the people of color and other disadvantaged groups have access to a lesser or zero health care. The case of *Plessy v. Ferguson* introduced the phrase "separate but equal" as well as State-endorsed racial segregation laws for public facilities, the reverberations of which persevere to the present day. Hence, the health-care system was characterized by de jure segregation (legal segregation) from 1865 through 1965, which, among other things, kept health care separate between Blacks and Whites, and de facto segregation (illegal segregation) currently prevails, where legislation does not openly segregate communities of color from gaining access to quality health-care equivalent to that of Whites, but, nonetheless, de facto health-care segregation persists.

Clearly then, American Indians and Blacks, and subsequently, other people of color, continue to live perpetually within a culture of segregation and persisting health disparities, within or without a pandemic. Health disparities are differences in health, where the socially disadvantaged (the poor, racial/ethnic minorities, women, and other groups, who remain enduringly susceptible to social disadvantage or discrimination) systematically face poorer health or more health risks than advantaged social groups. Any process to purge health disparities necessitates pursuing health equity (Braveman, 2006), which would demand ending systemic racism, poverty, and discrimination among Blacks and other people of color.

Racial health disparities represent a barrier to prevent people of color from receiving appropriate care as and when required to protect themselves from contracting the highly transmissible COVID-19 and other infections. Universal health care can dampen the effect of racial health disparities through ensuring that no one is prevented from receiving care, due to unaffordable out-of-pocket costs (Smith, 2020). But universal health care is not the reality in the USA. So who are the uninsured? In 2018, there were some 27.9 million uninsured Americans, increasing by about 500,000 from 2017, where the majority of the uninsured were from low-income families with at least one worker in the family. The communities of color were at greater risk of being uninsured than Whites and were at high risk of experiencing major health conditions and contracting chronic diseases (Tolbert et al., 2019). About 51% of the uninsured are Blacks or Hispanics (Smith, 2020), who, by virtue of their "uninsured" status, may be more probable to postpone COVID-19 testing and treatment, placing uninsured Blacks and other people of color at high risk. So how do we efficaciously reduce or eliminate this problem of vulnerability of Blacks and other people of color to contracting diseases and other illnesses? Byrd and Clayton (2012) argued that health problems experienced by Blacks are part of the structure and culture of the US health system. Thus, they argued that while health promotion and disease prevention and correction to the race-based socioeconomic problems are the way forward, they are insufficient; and that a better approach would require an equalization of the health delivery system, which eventually could dilute the impact of segregation. And so, presenting the major poor health outcomes in the USA is a powerful illustration of how race and class-based segregation of healthcare impacts Blacks and other communities of color; and which could point the way forward toward addressing racial health disparities.

Poor Health Outcomes

Hardly anyone can fault the USA on being meager with spending on health care. For some years now, the USA has incurred huge national health expenditures as a percentage of the gross domestic product (GDP), with 18% in 2020 (Keehan et al., 2020). US health expenditures are higher than their developed counterparts because it spends more on general practitioners' salaries, pharmaceuticals, and health-care administration (Papanicolas et al., 2018): for example, the US general practitioner's salary is US$ 218,173, twice the average salary across all high-income countries; specialists and nurses in the USA also earn higher salaries than other countries; on pharmaceuticals, the USA spends US$ 1443 per person, compared to the average of US$749 in other high-income countries; the USA expends 8% of total national health expenditures on planning, regulating, and managing health systems and services, compared to an average 3% among high-income countries. Despite lower health expenditures than the USA, advanced countries have attained better health outcomes for their people. Table 1.1 presents evidence from the USA, G7 nations,

Table 1.1 Health indices, selected OECD countries (6), 2018

Country	Health care as a percentage of GDP, 2019 (1)	Maternal mortality rate (deaths per 100,000 live births), 2018	Infant mortality rate (deaths per 1000 live births), 2018	Female life expectancy at birth (years), 2018	Male life expectancy at birth (years), 2018	Deaths per 100,000 population, standardized rates, 2017
Australia	9.3	4.8	3.1	84.9	80.7	634.4
Austria	10.4	7.1	2.7	84.1	79.4	741.4
Belgium	10.3	5 (7)	3.8	83.9	79.4	11 (5)
Canada (G7)	10.8	8.6	4.7	84.1	79.9	668.6
Denmark	10.0	1.6	3.7	82.9	79.1	10 (5)
Finland	9.1	4.2	2.1	84.5	79.1	729.1
France (G7)	11.2	8 (7)	3.8	85.9	79.7	9 (5)
Germany (G7)	11.7	3.2	3.2	83.3	78.6	780.5
Italy (G7)	8.7	2 (7)	2.0.8	85.6	81.2	11 (5)
Japan(G7)	11.1	3.6	1.9	87.3 (4)	81.1 (4)	562
New Zealand	9.3		3.8 (2)	83.5	80	7 (5)
Norway	10.5	1.8	2.3	84.5	81.1	8 (5)
Sweden	10.9	4.3	2	84.3	80.9	707
Switzerland	12.1	5 (7)	3.3	85.7	81.9	8 (5)
United Kingdom (G7)	10.3	7 (7)	3.9	83.1	79.5	9 (5)
United States (G7)	17.0	17.4	5.7 (3)	81.2	76.2	840.2

Source: OECD (2021b). Health Status [Online]. https://stats.oecd.org/Index. aspx?DataSetCode=HEALTH_STAT (Accessed August 4, 2021)
Notes
(1) OECD (2021a). Health expenditure and financing [Online]. https://stats.oecd.org/Index. aspx?DataSetCode=SHA (Accessed August 4, 2021)
(2) New Zealand Government (2019)
(3) CDC (2020)
(4) 2017
(5) Per 1000 people; 2018; (World Bank, 2019a)
(6) OECD countries: Australia, Austria, Belgium, Canada, Chile, Colombia, Czech Republic, Denmark, Estonia, Finland, France, Germany, Greece, Hungary, Iceland, Ireland, Israel, Italy, Japan, Korea, Latvia, Lithuania, Luxembourg, Mexico, the Netherlands, New Zealand, Norway, Poland, Portugal, Slovak Republic, Slovenia, Spain, Sweden, Switzerland, Turkey, United Kingdom, United States of America
(7) World Bank (2019b)
Maternal mortality ratio (modeled estimate, per 100,000 live births) for 2017

and selected OECD countries on infant mortality, life expectancy, maternal mortality, and death rate, to show the poor health outcomes in the USA, particularly among people of color, despite huge US health expenditures.

Life Expectancy

Life expectancy at birth is defined as how long a newborn may expect to live, assuming the prevailing death rates do not change. Table 1.1 shows that in 2018, the USA had a female life expectancy at birth of 81.2, and among the 37 OECD countries, inclusive of the G7 nations, only Mexico (77.9) had a lower female life expectancy than the USA (see full table at (OECD, 2021b)). Again in 2018, the USA had a male life expectancy at birth of 76.2, the lowest among the G7 countries (Canada, France, Germany, Italy, Japan, UK, and the USA). In the USA in 2017, the life expectancy at birth in years for White females was 81.0, White males 76.1; Black females 78.1, Black males 71.5; and Hispanic females 84.3, Hispanic males 79.1 (CDC, 2018). In 2017, compared to other race/ethnic groups in the US, Blacks had the lowest life expectancy at birth for both females and males.

Maternal Mortality

Maternal mortality rate is defined as the death of a woman during pregnancy, at delivery, or soon after delivery. Table 1.1 shows that in 2018, the USA had a maternal mortality rate of 17.4 per 100,000 live births, the highest among the G7 countries and the 37 OECD countries, except Mexico (see full table at (OECD, 2021b)). In the USA in 2019, maternal mortality rates per 100,000 live births by race/ethnicity were as follows: Whites 17.9, Blacks 44.0, and Hispanics 12.6. In 2019, compared to other race/ethnic groups in the US, Blacks had the highest maternal mortality rate (Hoyert, 2020).

Death Rate

The death rate is the frequency of occurrence of death in a specific population over a specified period. Table 1.1 shows that in 2017, the USA had 840.2 deaths per 100,000 people, the highest among the selected OECD countries inclusive of the G7 nations, with Japan recording the lowest at 562 per 100,000 live births (see full table at (OECD, 2021b)). The age-adjusted death rates per 100,000 by race and ethnicity in 2017 in the USA were as follows: non-Hispanic White population, 755.0 deaths; non-Hispanic Black population, 881.0; and Hispanic population, 524.7; the age-adjusted death rate has been 1.2 times greater for non-Hispanic Blacks than for the non-Hispanic Whites since 2008, and the rate has been 1.4 times greater for non-Hispanic Whites than for Hispanics with no change since 2010. The racial mortality gap remains sizable, with life expectancies in 2018 for non-Hispanic Black females and non-Hispanic Black males 3.1 years and 4.9 years lower than non-Hispanic White females and males, respectively (NCHS and CDC, 2020). The variance in the racial mortality gap was characteristic of the 50 States of the USA (NCHS and CDC, 2017).

Cancer

A review of cancer reveals the nature of racial health disparities (Siegel et al., 2020). Generally, cancer incidence rates had been highest among Whites, due to the high rate of lung cancer and female breast cancer. But, sex-specific incidence was at its peak in Black men from 2012 through 2016, where it was 85% greater than those in Asian/Pacific Islander men, who have the lowermost rates, and 8% greater than those in White men, who were placed second. Among women, Whites had the peak incidence rate, 8% higher than Blacks, who were placed second. Nevertheless, Black women had the highest cancer mortality rates – 13% greater than those for White women. The mortality disparity among men was similarly greater, with the death rate in Black men two times that of Asian/Pacific Islander men and 20% higher than that in White men. Nonetheless, the Black-White disparity in overall cancer mortality among men and women together dropped from a peak of 33% in 1993 to 13% in 2017. There was a steep drop in deaths in smoking-related cancers among Blacks, as there was a sharp decline in smoking prevalence (Siegel et al., 2020). Siegel et al. (2018) presented data in previous years showing that in 2015, Blacks experienced a 14% higher cancer death rate than Whites, the racial disparity was greater for those aged <65 years compared with those aged ≥65 years, and the racial disparity was different significantly by State.

Cardiovascular Disease

Cardiovascular disease or heart disease, the leading cause of death in the USA in 2019, accounted for 659,041 deaths (NCHS/CDC, 2021). Deaths per 100,000 among race/ethnic groups in 2017 were as follows: White 168.9, Black 208.0, and Hispanic 114.1 (CDC, 2019b). The 2017 National Health Interview Survey (Virani et al., 2020) showed that the age-adjusted prevalence of different types of heart disease was 10.6%, and the age-adjusted prevalence rates of heart disease among race/ethnic groups were as follows: Whites 11.0%, Blacks 9.7%, and Hispanics 7.4%, and the age-adjusted prevalence of heart disease, coronary artery disease, hypertension, and stroke was greater in males (11.8%, 7.2%, 26.0%, and 3.3%, correspondingly) than females (9.5%, 4.2%, 23.1%, and 2.5%, correspondingly). Cardiovascular health disparities between Blacks and Whites remain a major disease burden in American life and as the leading cause of death involving some 85.6 million Americans (Tabb et al., 2020). The study (Tabb et al., 2020) concluded that there were substantial Black-White racial disparities in cardiovascular health, with Blacks constantly having worse total cardiovascular health scores in relation to Whites.

Black Women and Reproductive Health

Black women's sexual exploitation and health-care disenfranchisement are well-known in American history. Prather et al. (2018) discussed how Black women's sexual and reproductive health has been compromised as a result of their manifold experiences of racism as well as discriminatory health-care practices from slavery through the post-Civil Rights era, ultimately impacting contemporary epidemiology of their sexual and reproductive health disparities. Black women faced disproportionate pregnancy-related morbidity and mortality (Dominguez, 2011; Aziz & Smith, 2011). For instance, in 2013, the preterm rate for Black infants was approximately 60% greater than that for White infants (17.1% and 10.8%, correspondingly) (Martin et al., 2013). Moreover, the low birth weight rate for Black infants was 10.13% and 6.97% for Whites (Martin et al., 2003). Furthermore, compared to other women, through 1998–2005, Black women carried a three to four times greater risk of pregnancy-related death, for pregnancy-related hypertension and chronic hypertension (Martin et al., 2011), and the least likely to be recipient of prenatal care (Tucker et al., 2007). In 2019, maternal deaths per 100,000 live births among Black women were 44.0, White 17.9, and Hispanics 12.6 (Hoyert, 2020).

HIV/AIDS

Blacks have long since been overrepresented in HIV/AIDS, a disparity that has expanded over the years. In 2018, Blacks constituted 13% of the population, but comprised 42% (16,002) of the 37,968 new HIV diagnoses, mostly among Blacks; toward the end of 2018, the USA had 1.2 million people living with HIV, of which 482,900 were Black; in 2018, six (6) in seven (7) of Blacks were aware of their HIV status, and 6678 deaths occurred among Blacks diagnosed with HIV in the USA (CDC, 2021).

Discussion

The "in search of a new whole-of-society paradigm" is hotly being pursued for explanations because of the failure of huge US health expenditures to deliver better health outcomes for all Americans and also the failure to wipe out racial health disparities. Nonetheless, financial resources may be necessary but not sufficient to address the problem of racial health disparities. After 401 years (1619–2020) of slavery, Black Codes/Jim Crow, Ku Klux Klan episodes, Civil Rights, and post-Civil Rights, the disparity in health outcomes between the Black and White populations remains a plague in American public health. Such health disparities also afflict Hispanics, American Indians/Alaska Natives (AI/AN), Asian Americans, and other ethnic minority groups. But what is the reason for this perpetual prevalence of poor health outcomes and racial health disparities inflicted against Blacks and the poor? Perhaps, the health-care system should develop more preventive measures as having better social value than curative treatments and that health is really an outcome of social and economic organization. This approach would induce greater utility than compulsively focusing on clinical treatment. Government authorities should be focusing more on health promotion, disease prevention, and prolonging life, in order to achieve a state of physical and mental well-being for all its people. For instance,

> Achieving and maintaining health are not just matters of curing illness. The ways in which society regulates employment and economic cycles, provides education, assists its members in times of economic and other difficulties, sets up strategies to counteract poverty, crime, and drug abuse and to stimulate economic and social growth have just as much, if not more, impact on health than do the quantity and quality of resources being invested in the detection and care of illness (Renaud, 1994, p. 318).

At the dawn of the twentieth century, Du Bois refuted the view that preoccupations and responsibilities with illness care would lead to the demise of diseases and sicknesses. Throughout the years 1901–1903, death rates for pneumonia (inflammation of the lungs) among Blacks were higher than those for Whites. Reviewing deaths from 17 out of about 50 diseases showed that Blacks were demographically overrepresented (Du Bois, 2003). In fact, Du Bois also was among the first to document that health disparities of African Americans compared to Whites in the country emanated from social conditions and not from racial traits and tendencies, and should there be better sanitary conditions, better education, and improved economic opportunities, their mortality may decline and become normal (Du Bois, 2003).

But this notion of social and economic conditions as key determinants of health was not new. The Greek philosopher Plato (2010) argued that income and wealth distribution was critical to prevent plagues vis-à-vis his legislative proposal of no extreme poverty and no excess wealth. Engels (2008) in the mid-nineteenth-century England showed the link between working conditions and health and the political and economic systems that generated conditions resulting in health inequalities. He felt that people living in deplorable conditions would experience poor health and low life expectancy. Then there was Virchow (1848), reporting in 1848 on the typhus epidemic in Upper Silesia, and who stated that diseases were always traceable to societal defects. One of those societal defects would be systemic racism.

White-imposed racism has remained a major perpetual contributor to racial and ethnic inequalities along with health inequities, where delivering health care means delivering illness care. Therefore, it is not surprising that throughout American history, epidemic diseases have exacted a demographically disproportionate toll on Blacks and Indigenous people, and later, on other communities of color. It may very well be the case that the obligations and concerns of Departments/Ministries of Health are heavily influenced by illness care. And "If they were actually responsible for health, their main concern would be to improve the social and economic conditions that affect the individuals' ability to make health-enhancing life-style decisions and to react and respond calmly to life's inevitable problems" (Renaud, 1994, p. 318). Hence, Blacks and other communities of color continuously suffer poor health outcomes, rooted in systemic racism. Health-care improvements for the people of color who are really the poor and vulnerable require betterment in their social and economic conditions to generate better health decisions, health equity, and eventually bettering population health. The following data shows the racist realities and outcomes of the major institutions of US society:

In the third quarter of 2020 for persons 16 years and older, the unemployment rates by race and ethnicity (BLS, 2020) were as follows: Blacks at 13.2% and Hispanics at 11.2% compared to Whites at 7.9%. In 2019, Blacks comprised 13.2% of the total population in the USA but 23.8% of the poverty population and Hispanics comprised 18.7% of the total population but 28.1% of the poverty population (Creamer, 2020). In 2019, the median household income for Black households was US$ 45,438, US$ 56,113 for Hispanic households, and US$ 76,057 for non-Hispanic White households (Creamer, 2020). In 2017, non-Hispanic White households had a median household wealth of US$ 171,700, US$ 9567 for Black households, and US$ 25,000 for Hispanic households (Hays & Sullivan, 2020). In 2019 (Beyer, 2020), 42% of Black families and 73% of Whites were homeowners, but 49% of Blacks were homeowners in 2004. The housing crisis in 2008 hit Black homeowners very severely, where some 70% Black households probably experienced foreclosure than White households. Even after many years of the Fair Housing Act of 1968, which outlawed discrimination in housing sales, rentals, or financing based on religion, race, or national origin, residential segregation is still extensive in the USA (Beyer, 2020). Through the 51 metropolitan areas in the USA with no less than 1 million residents, the average segregation index still hovered at almost 60, where 0 signifies full integration and 100 denotes complete separation of racial groups.

Notwithstanding that the Civil Rights laws of the 1960s ended Jim Crow, US policy and legal responses have done precious little to end the growing racial health disparities along with the devastating and disproportionate COVID-19 impact on people of color. There is possibly now a new Jim Crow framework (Alexander, 2020; Massey, 2007). Thus, we should remind ourselves "…that slavery was at bottom a social arrangement, a way of society's ordering its members in its own mind" (Jordan, 1962 p. 30). This stratified social arrangement/racial hierarchy predated

COVID-19, whereby it presented a persisting culture of racial/ethnic inequalities historically rooted in slavery, was intergenerational, as well as part of the culture (Bowser, 2017). Therefore, with racial stratification powering society, it is hard to visualize policy responses for COVID-19 as a game changer for ending racism and the onslaught of this pandemic on communities of color.

The poor health outcomes on infant mortality rate, life expectancy, death rate, maternal mortality, cancer, cardiovascular diseases, reproductive issues, and HIV/AIDS have exacted a demographically disproportionate toll on Blacks and Indigenous people, and later, on other communities of color, where all their health outcomes have roots in systemic racism. Over the years, numerous research findings have signaled a significant US public health problem containing systemic racism against all racial groups, particularly people of color (Feagin & Bennefield, 2014). Race and class-based segregation of health care and racial health disparities constitute a public health crisis and remain a pestilence in the American healthcare system, and now, the new Jim Crow environment has emerged. Likewise, the failure of huge US health expenditures to deliver better health outcomes for all Americans becomes a compelling dynamic to understand how this country has been managing COVID-19 through reviewing the epidemiology of this pathogen.

References

Alexander, M. (2020). *The new Jim crow: Mass incarceration in the age of colorblindness*. The New Press.

Arnold, C. (2018). *Pandemic 1918: Eyewitness accounts from the greatest medical holocaust in modern history*. St. Martin's Press.

Aziz, M., & Smith, K. Y. (2011). Challenges and successes in linking HIV-infected women to care in the United States. *Clinical Infectious Diseases, 52*, S231–S237.

Beyer, D. (2020). *The economic state of black America in 2020* [online]. Joint Economic Committee. U.S. Congress. Available: https://www.jec.senate.gov/public/_cache/files/ccf4dbe2-810a-44f8-b3e7-14f7e5143ba6/economic-state-of-black-america-2020.pdf. Accessed 2 Dec 2020.

BLS. (2020). *Labor Force Statistics from the Current Population Survey* [Online]. Available: https://www.bls.gov/web/empsit/cpsee_e16.htm. Accessed 2 Dec 2020.

Bond, J. (1997). Preface. In C., H. (Ed.), *Double exposure: Poverty and race in America*. M.E Sharp.

Bowser, B. P. (2017). Racism: Origin and theory. *Journal of Black Studies, 48*, 572–590.

Braveman, P. (2006). Health disparities and health equity: Concepts and measurement. *Annual Review of Public Health, 27*, 167–194.

Byrd, W. M., & Clayton, L. A. (1992). An American health dilemma: A history of blacks in the health system. *Journal of the National Medical Association, 84*, 189.

Byrd, W. M., & Clayton, L. A. (2012). *An American health dilemma: A medical history of African Americans and the problem of race: Beginnings to 1900*. Routledge.

CDC. (2018). Table 4. Life expectancy at birth, at age 65, and at age 75, by sex, race, and Hispanic origin: United States, selected years 1900–2017. *NCHS*.

CDC. (2019a). *1918 Pandemic (H1N1 virus)* [online]. CDC. Available: https://www.cdc.gov/flu/pandemic-resources/1918-pandemic-h1n1.html. Accessed 31 July 2021.

CDC. (2019b). *Racial and ethnic disparities in heart disease* [online]. CDC. Available: https://www.cdc.gov/nchs/hus/spotlight/2019-heart-disease-disparities.htm. Accessed 9 Aug 2021.

CDC. (2020). *Reproductive health* [Online]. CDC. Available: https://www.cdc.gov/reproductive-health/maternalinfanthealth/infantmortality.htm. Accessed 4 Aug 2021.

CDC. (2021). *HIV and African American people* [online]. CDC. Available: https://www.cdc.gov/hiv/group/racialethnic/africanamericans/index.html. Accessed 27 June 2021.

Creamer, J. (2020). *Inequalities persist despite decline in poverty for all major race and Hispanic origin groups* [Online]. United states census bureau. Available: https://www.census.gov/library/stories/2020/09/poverty-rates-for-blacks-and-hispanics-reached-historic-lows-in-2019.html. Accessed 2 Dec 2020.

Cunningham, T. J., Croft, J. B., Liu, Y., Lu, H., Eke, P. I., & Giles, W. H. (2017). Vital signs: Racial disparities in age-specific mortality among blacks or African Americans—United States, 1999–2015. *MMWR. Morbidity and Mortality Weekly Report, 66,* 444.

De Beauvoir, S. (2010). *The second sex.* Knopf.

Dominguez, T. P. (2011). Adverse birth outcomes in African American women: The social context of persistent reproductive disadvantage. *Social Work in Public Health, 26,* 3–16.

Du Bois, W. B. (2003). The health and physique of the negro American. *American Journal of Public Health, 93,* 272–276.

Engels, F. (2008). *The condition of the working class in England in 1844.* Cosimo.

Feagin, J. R. (2020). *The white racial frame: Centuries of racial framing and counter-framing.* Routledge.

Feagin, J., & Bennefield, Z. (2014). Systemic racism and US health care. *Social Science & Medicine, 103,* 7–14.

Fields, E. L., Copeland, R., & Hopkins, E. (2021). Same script, different viruses: HIV and COVID-19 in US black communities. *The Lancet, 397,* 1040–1042.

Gaskin, D. J., Arbelaez, J. J., Brown, J. R., Petras, H., Wagner, F. A., & Cooper, L. A. (2007). Examining racial and ethnic disparities in site of usual source of care. *Journal of the National Medical Association, 99,* 22.

Gaskin, D. J., Dinwiddie, G. Y., Chan, K. S., & Mccleary, R. (2012a). Residential segregation and disparities in health care services utilization. *Medical Care Research and Review, 69,* 158–175.

Gaskin, D. J., Dinwiddie, G. Y., Chan, K. S., & Mccleary, R. R. (2012b). Residential segregation and the availability of primary care physicians. *Health Services Research, 47,* 2353–2376.

Gaskin, D. J., Dinwiddie, G. Y., Chan, K. S., & Mccleary, R. R. (2012c). Residential segregation and the availability of primary care physicians. *Health Services Research, 47,* 2353–2376.

GLL. (2020a). *A Brief History of Civil Rights in the United States* [Online]. Available: https://guides.ll.georgetown.edu/c.php?g=592919&p=4172697. Accessed 23 Jan 2021.

GLL. (2020b). *A Brief History of Civil Rights in the United States* [Online]. Available: https://guides.ll.georgetown.edu/c.php?g=592919&p=4172700. Accessed 22 Jan 2021.

Godlee, F., & Silberner, J. (2020). The BMJ interview: Anthony Fauci on covid-19. *BMJ, 370,* m3703.

Greene, J., Blustein, J., & Weitzman, B. C. (2006). Race, segregation, and physicians' participation in Medicaid. *The Milbank Quarterly, 84,* 239–272.

Hammonds, E. M., & Reverby, S. M. (2019). *Toward a historically informed analysis of racial health disparities since 1619.* American Public Health Association.

Hays, D. & Sullivan, B. (2020). *2017 Data Show Homeowners Nearly 89 Times Wealthier Than Renters* [Online]. Available: https://www.census.gov/library/stories/2020/11/gaps-in-wealth-of-americans-by-household-type-in-2017.html. Accessed 2 Dec 2020.

Hoyert, D. L. (2020). *Maternal mortality rates in the United States, 2019.*

JHU CSSE. (2021). *COVID-19 dashboard* [online]. Johns Hopkins University & Medicine Coronavirus Resource Center. Available: https://coronavirus.jhu.edu/map.html. Accessed 2 Aug 2021.

Jordan, W. D. (1962). Modern tensions and the origins of American slavery. *The Journal of Southern History, 28,* 18–30.

Keehan, S. P., Cuckler, G. A., Poisal, J. A., Sisko, A. M., Smith, S. D., Madison, A. J., Rennie, K. E., Fiore, J. A., & Hardesty, J. C. (2020). National Health Expenditure Projections, 2019–28:

Expected rebound in prices drives rising spending growth: National health expenditure projections for the period 2019–2028. *Health Affairs, 39*, 704–714.

Kirby, J. B., & Kaneda, T. (2005). Neighborhood socioeconomic disadvantage and access to health care. *Journal of Health and Social Behavior, 46*, 15–31.

Krieger, N., Rehkopf, D. H., Chen, J. T., Waterman, P. D., Marcelli, E., & Kennedy, M. (2008). The fall and rise of US inequities in premature mortality: 1960–2002. *PLoS Medicine, 5*, e46.

Martin, J. A., Hamilton, B. E., Sutton, P. D., Ventura, S. J., Menacker, F., & Munson, M. L. (2003). Births: Final data for 2002. *National Vital Statistics Reports, 52*, 1–113.

Martin, J. A., Hamilton, B. E., Ventura, S. J., Osterman, M. J., Kirmeyer, S., Mathews, T., & Wilson, E. C. (2011). *Births: Final data for 2009* (Vol. 60, pp. 1–70). National vital statistics reports: from the Centers for Disease Control and Prevention, National Center for Health Statistics, National Vital Statistics System.

Martin, J. A., Osterman, M., Control, C. F. D., & PREVENTION. (2013). Preterm births—United States, 2006 and 2010. *MMWR Surveillance Summaries, 62*, 136–138.

Massey, D. S. (2007). *Categorically unequal: The American stratification system*. Russell Sage Foundation.

Massey, D. S., & Fischer, M. J. (2000). How segregation concentrates poverty. *Ethnic and Racial Studies, 23*, 670–691.

Massey, D. S., & Fong, E. (1990). Segregation and neighborhood quality: Blacks, Hispanics, and Asians in the San Francisco metropolitan area. *Social Forces, 69*, 15–32.

Massey, D. S., Gross, A. B., & Eggers, M. L. (1991). Segregation, the concentration of poverty, and the life chances of individuals. *Social Science Research, 20*, 397–420.

Matthew, D. B. (2018). *Just medicine: A cure for racial inequality in American health care*. NYU Press.

National Academies of Sciences, E. & Medicine. (2017). *Communities in action: Pathways to health equity*.

NCHS & CDC. (2017). *Table 16. Age-adjusted death rates, by race, Hispanic origin, state, and territory: United States and U.S. dependent areas, average annual* 1979–1981, *1989–1991, and 2014–2016* [Online]. Available: https://www.cdc.gov/nchs/data/hus/2017/016.pdf. Accessed 27 Nov 2020.

NCHS & CDC. (2020). *United States Life Tables, 2018* [Online]. Available: https://www.cdc.gov/nchs/data/nvsr/nvsr69/nvsr69-12-508.pdf. Accessed 26 Nov 2020.

NCHS/CDC. (2021). *Heart disease* [online]. NCHS/CDC. Available: https://www.cdc.gov/nchs/fastats/heart-disease.htm. Accessed 6 June 2021.

New Zealand Government. (2019). *Infant mortality rate declines* [online]. New Zealand Government. Available: https://www.stats.govt.nz/news/infant-mortality-rate-declines. Accessed 4 Aug 2021.

NYT. (2021). *Biden's speech to congress: Full transcript* [online]. The New York Times. Available: https://www.nytimes.com/2021/04/29/us/politics/joe-biden-speech-transcript.html. Accessed 9 Aug 2021.

ODPHP. (2021). *Disparities* [Online]. ODPHP, DHHS. Available: https://www.healthypeople.gov/2020/about/foundation-health-measures/Disparities. Accessed 23 May 2021.

OECD. (2021a). *Health expenditure and financing* [online]. OECD. Available: https://stats.oecd.org/Index.aspx?DataSetCode=SHA. Accessed 4 Aug 2021.

OECD. (2021b). *Health status* [online]. OECD. Available: https://stats.oecd.org/Index.aspx?DataSetCode=HEALTH_STAT. Accessed 4 Aug 2021.

Papanicolas, I., Woskie, L. R., & Jha, A. K. (2018). Health care spending in the United States and other high-income countries. *JAMA, 319*, 1024–1039.

PLATO. (2010). *The Laws: Books 1–6* [Online]. Available: http://www.greektexts.com/library/plato/laws_(books_1_-_6)/eng/317.html. Accessed 8 Dec 2020.

Prather, C., Fuller, T. R., Jeffries, W. L., IV, Marshall, K. J., Howell, A. V., Belyue-Umole, A., & King, W. (2018). Racism, African American women, and their sexual and reproductive health:

A review of historical and contemporary evidence and implications for health equity. *Health equity, 2*, 249–259.

Renaud, M. (1994). The future: Hygeia versus Panakeia? In R. G. Evans, M. L. Barer, & T. R. Marmor (Eds.), *Why are some people healthy and others not? The determinants of health of populations*. Aldine De Gruyter.

Roberts, D. (2011). *Fatal invention: How science, politics, and big business re-create race in the twenty-first century*. New Press/ORIM.

Siegel, R. L., Miller, K. D., & Jemal, A. (2018). Cancer statistics, 2018. *CA: a Cancer Journal for Clinicians, 68*, 7–30.

Siegel, R. L., Miller, K. D., & Jemal, A. (2020). Cancer statistics, 2020. *CA: a Cancer Journal for Clinicians, 70*, 7–30.

Smith, D. B. (2020). The pandemic challenge: End separate and unequal healthcare. *The American Journal of the Medical Sciences, 360*, 109–111.

Tabb, L. P., Ortiz, A., Judd, S., Cushman, M., & Mcclure, L. A. (2020). Exploring the spatial patterning in racial differences in cardiovascular health between blacks and whites across the United States: The REGARDS study. *Journal of the American Heart Association, 9*, e016556.

Tolbert, J., Orgera, K., Singer, N. & Damico, A. (2019). *Key Facts about the Uninsured Population* [Online]. Available: http://files.kff.org/attachment//fact-sheet-key-facts-about-the-uninsured-population. Accessed 24 Jan 2021.

Tucker, M. J., Berg, C. J., Callaghan, W. M., & Hsia, J. (2007). The black–white disparity in pregnancy-related mortality from 5 conditions: Differences in prevalence and case-fatality rates. *American Journal of Public Health, 97*, 247–251.

U.S.C. (1964). *Title VI of the civil rights act of 1964* [online]. U.S. Department of Justice. Available: https://www.govinfo.gov/content/pkg/USCODE-2010-title42/pdf/USCODE-2010-title42-chap21-subchapV.pdf. Accessed 30 Mar 2021.

USCB. (2012). *Statistical abstract of the United States: 2012. Table 168. Ambulatory care visits to physicians' offices and hospital outpatient and emergency departments: 2008.* [online]. U.S. Department of Commerce: USCB. Available: http://www.census.gov/compendia/statab/2012/tables/12s0168.pdf. Accessed 6 Mar 2021.

USDHHS. (1985–1986). *Report of the Secretary's Task Force on Black & Minority Health* [Online]. Available: https://www.minorityhealth.hhs.gov/assets/pdf/checked/1/ANDERSON.pdf. Accessed 29 Jan 2021.

USNCHS. (2012). *National health statistics reports; ambulatory care visits to physicians' offices. 2003.* [online]. CDC. Available: www.census.gov/compendia/statab/2012/tables/12s0168.xls. Accessed 6 Mar 2021.

Virani, S. S., Alonso, A., Benjamin, E. J., Bittencourt, M. S., Callaway, C. W., Carson, A. P., Chamberlain, A. M., Chang, A. R., Cheng, S., Delling, F. N., Djousse, L., Elkind, M. S. V., Ferguson, J. F., Fornage, M., Khan, S. S., Kissela, B. M., Knutson, K. L., Kwan, T. W., Lackland, D. T., … Tsao, C. W. (2020). Heart Disease and Stroke Statistics—2020 Update: A report From the American Heart Association. *Circulation, 141*, e139–e596.

Virchow, R. (1848). *Report on the Typhus Epidemic in Upper Silesia*.

World Bank. (2019a). *Death rate, crude (per 1,000 people)* [online]. World Bank. Available: https://data.worldbank.org/indicator/SP.DYN.CDRT.IN?locations=BE. Accessed 4 Aug 2021.

World Bank. (2019b). *Maternal mortality ratio (modeled estimate, per 100,000 live births)* [online]. World Bank. Available: https://data.worldbank.org/indicator/SH.STA.MMRT. Accessed 5 Aug 2021.

Yancy, C. W. (2020). COVID-19 and African Americans. *JAMA, 323*(19), 1891–1892. https://doi.org/10.1001/jama.2020.6548

Chapter 2
Epidemiology of COVID-19

Beginnings of COVID-19

Pandemics seem to emerge in threesome per century (Sandman, 2007); and the twentieth century brought the severe "Spanish Flu" with A (H1N1) virus in 1918–1919, then the milder "Asian flu" with A (H2N2) virus in 1957–1958, followed by the mildest "Hong Kong Flu" with A (H3N2) virus in 1968–1969. The powerful modern global transportation and communication technology in the twentieth century guaranteed a rapid viral transmission of these diseases. Then in the first two decades of the twenty-first century, two novel coronavirus outbreaks occurred. First, there was the outbreak of SARS in 2002–2003 caused by SARS-CoV, which carried a case fatality rate of about 10% (8098 confirmed cases and 774 deaths); the second was MERS caused by MERS-CoV, with a case fatality rate of 34.4% (2502 confirmed cases and 861 deaths) between April 2012 and December 2019 (Park, 2020).

Then a new coronavirus contagion hit China on December 12, 2019. Several cases emerged caused by an unidentified pneumonia disease that originated from a local seafood market in Wuhan City, Hubei Province of China. By January 26, 2020, the number of infections grew to 2761 in China with 80 deaths, and 33 infected people in 10 other countries (WMHC, 2020). Characteristic clinical symptoms of these patients were fever, dry cough, breathing problems (dyspnea), headache, and pneumonia (Zhou et al., 2020). The samples of seven patients with severe pneumonia (six sellers or deliverymen from the seafood market) (Zhou et al., 2020) at the intensive care unit of Wuhan Jin Yin-Tan Hospital at the commencement of the outbreak were referred to the laboratory at the Wuhan Institute of Virology (WIV) for diagnosis of the causative agent, but two of them were discharged; the remaining five samples indicated positivity for coronaviruses, where 87.1% sequences matched the SARS-related coronaviruses; then Zhou et al. indicated that full-length genome sequences of 2019-novel coronavirus (2019-nCOV) (named after the WHO referred to this virus as novel coronavirus) were extracted for four samples, and they were

99.9% identical to each other, and additional analysis showed that some of the 2019-nCoV genes carried less than 80% nucleotide sequence identity to SARS-CoV. But the analysis also showed that their amino acid sequences used for coronavirus species classification were 94.4% identical between 2019nCov and SARS-CoV, demonstrating that the two viruses matched the same species severe acute respiratory syndrome-related coronavirus (SARSr-CoV) (Zhou et al., 2020).

The WHO China Country Office on December 31, 2019, was informed about these pneumonia cases of unknown etiology identified in Wuhan City, China. Afterwards, from December 31, 2019 through January 3, 2020, a collection of 44 cases of severe pneumonia of unknown etiology was reported to the WHO by China. On January 8, 2020, the Coronavirus Study Group (CSG) of the International Committee on Taxonomy of Viruses (ICTV) identified and labeled this virus as SARS-CoV-2, the virus that causes COVID-19. The SARS-CoV-2 employs the same host receptor, angiotensin-converting enzyme 2 (ACE2), as that utilized by SARS-CoV to infect humans (ICTV, 2020), with human-to-human transmission via airborne droplet reported shortly thereafter. The WHO on January 11 and 12, 2020, obtained additional information from the China National Health Commission that the outbreak was linked to exposures in one seafood market in Wuhan City and that the Chinese authorities recognized a new type of coronavirus, which was isolated on January 7, 2020. Then on January 12, 2020, China shared the genetic sequence of the novel coronavirus to enable other countries to build specific diagnostic kits. The WHO officially declared COVID-19 as a pandemic on March 11, 2020, due to its scale and rapidity of transmission.

The USA confirmed the first case of 2019-nCoV in Washington State on January 21, 2020. This infected patient had returned from Wuhan, China, on January 15, 2020. Then US President Donald Trump declared a public health emergency vis-à-vis the Public Health Service Act on January 31, 2020. From its first case on January 21, 2020, the USA on May 24, 2021 (JHU, 2021), reached 33,120,470 cases and 589,925 deaths, and at May 24, 2021 (JHU, 2021), globally, the numbers totaled 167,261,131cases and 3,465,583 deaths. Undoubtedly, the contagion had then certainly arrived in the USA and had begun to increase its spread, unleashing a troubling impact on the society analogous only to the 1918 influenza pandemic, exposing and redefining persistent racial health disparities among the communities of color.

The WHO's declaration of COVID-19 as a pandemic was formalized virtually 3 months after its outbreak in Wuhan, China. At that juncture, the pathogen had already entered more than 114 countries, with 118,000 confirmed cases and some 4291 deaths. In fact, 2 weeks before the declaration of COVID-19 as a pandemic, cases increased 13-fold and countries impacted by the virus tripled (WHO, 2020c). If the COVID-19 had been declared a pandemic in January 2020, would that have made any difference to the US? Let us consider China's rapid response to COVID-19.

The China Experience

At the time of the of the COVID-19 outbreak, China initiated a rapid response (Liu et al., 2020), thus:

- December 29, 2019: China conducted an epidemiological investigation.
- January 1, 2020: South China seafood market in Wuhan was closed for business.
- January 23, 2020: Wuhan lockdown was executed.
- January 25, 2020: Communist Party of China (CPC) central committee established a prominent group to deal with the epidemic.
- Internet surveillance, involving Sina Weibo Index, Google Trends and Baidu Index, was utilized to monitor COVID-19.
- Epidemic prevention policies (strict restrictions on travel and public gatherings, closure of public places, implementation of strict temperature monitoring across the country, correct use of masks, suspension of work and school, personal monitoring at home, etc.). The Chinese population actively worked together.
- March 18, 2020: WHO representative in China, Dr. Colliers, explained that China has demonstrated that the trajectory of COVID-19 can be transformed.
- Characteristically, an epidemic develops exponentially, peaks, and then progressively starts to decline, when all susceptible people would have contracted the infection or became ill. Nonetheless, China did not exhibit that experience. The epidemiological curve in China was irregular, the epidemic was eliminated in its growth phase, and the spread of the virus was prevented. This Chinese experience reveals that not all infectious diseases need to become huge outbreaks, which may devastate health systems.
- March 19, 2020: zero new confirmed cases in China.

Important lessons from the China experience include early detection, early diagnosis, early quarantine, and early treatment. There is no question that early and rapid testing becomes critical in an outbreak, and the USA certainly was a laggard in the administration of testing.

Epidemiological Parameters on COVID-19 Transmission Dynamics

A comprehensive understanding of the spread of new COVID-19 infections in a timely fashion is necessary to evaluate the risks and the magnitude of this pandemic. As the virus spreads among the general population, public health authorities require reliable estimates of its transmission capability, the related uncertainties, and the influence of public health interventions (Xiang et al., 2021). In pursuing this task, we would need to describe the fundamental epidemiologic parameters.

In a situation where there is an unconstrained spread of the virus, the reproduction number of the virus referred to as R_0 ("R-nought"), indicating the number of people to whom an infected person can transmit the virus, lies within the range of 2 and 4 (Li et al., 2020c; Hao et al., 2020). A systematic review and meta-analysis based on 42 studies researched epidemiologic characteristics of SARS-CoV-2, the efficacy of control measures to apprise policymakers and leaders in framing management guidelines and to offer directions for future research (Park et al., 2020). This review found that estimates presented the reproduction number R_0 for this pandemic as 2.0–3.0, which provided a sense of the early epidemic spread, and was probably informative to public health authorities about the level of risk posed by COVID-19 and the impact of potential intervention strategies; this study also estimated the incubation period at 4–6 days, and the case fatality rate ranged from 0.3% to 1.4% for countries outside China.

According to Christakis (2020), the R_0 for both SARS and COVID-19 was within the range of 2.2–3.6. But the R_0 for SARS had a large variation, meaning it had a slower spread than COVID-19. SARs-CoV-2 has a higher spread in large clusters as seen in Wuhan's first outbreak (Salzberger et al., 2020), while household transmission rate was low (WHO, 2020a). Then there is the effective reproduction number, R_t, which shows the potential for epidemic spread at time t under the employment of prevention measures (Inglesby, 2020). Evaluating the effectiveness of public health interventions would necessitate the measurement of R_t in different environments and at regular intervals. Reduced social interactions can reduce R_t, which is reducing the spread. Inglesby (2020) noted that on January 23, 2020, the Chinese Government instituted in Wuhan a city lockdown and home and centralized quarantines, inclusive of total control of movements for months and compulsory isolation in facilities, as well as business closures, school closures, and a ban on gatherings, and where all worked to reduce the spread quite rapidly, bringing R_t to below 1. These measures have become the framework for social distancing interventions globally; and so, in the early phases of the pandemic without an effective vaccine, the appropriate public health goal involved employing a blend of these social distancing measures, in order to bring R_t to below 1.

The US study (Olney et al., 2020) of 29 States employed case fatalities from February 29, 2020, up to April 25, 2020, when some States commenced reversing their interventions used to stop the COVID-19 spread. The study assessed the effect of interventions across all the States, compared the estimated reproduction number, R_t, for each State before and after lockdown, and compared predicted upcoming fatalities with actual fatalities. This study found that lockdown and school closure as preventive measures to contain the spread have had the most reliable impact on R_t and lockdown seemed to have reduced R_t to below 1.0. However, lockdown was the least employed preventive intervention in the USA, so with a limited lockdown and no active enactment of additional preventive measures as social distancing, the transmission of SARS-CoV-2 continued (Olney et al., 2020). The study further noted that prior to a lockdown, none of the 29 States had an R_t below 1.0, but after lockdown, the States scored an R_t below 1.0. This study (Olney et al., 2020) concluded that in the absence of medical therapeutics and vaccines, social distancing still remains critical for limiting the spread.

It has become common knowledge among some people that COVID-19 symptoms are the same as the common cold. That said, controlling and containing the virus would then become problematic because of people's misguided and erroneous sense of the seriousness of the pandemic. So when do people identify the COVID-19 symptoms? Incubation is the period between contracting the infection and displaying symptoms, and this period ranges from 2 to 14 days for COVID-19, while the incubation period for SARS was 2–7 days, but it is the "latent period" (time between contracting the virus and transmitting this virus to other people), 1 day lesser than the incubation period (Salzberger et al., 2020), which marks a critical difference between SARS and COVID-19. And when the incubation and the latent periods are different, then that difference is referred to as the "mismatch period" (Christakis, 2020). There are more asymptomatic infected persons in a situation where the incubation period is longer than the latent period, as is the situation with COVID-19, making it more overwhelming than SARS (Christakis, 2020). The mismatch makes both SARS and COVID-19 differ in their spread, where COVID-19 may have a more rapid spread than SARS.

Serial interval refers to the time period from illness onset in the primary case to illness onset in the secondary case (Alene et al., 2021). The serial interval of infections at the beginning of the pandemic was estimated to be 7.6 days, but subsequently scaled down to about 4 days (Li et al. 2020b; Nishiura et al., 2020; Du et al., 2020). Alene et al. (2021), in their systematic review and meta-analysis of the serial interval and the incubation period of COVID-19, found the average serial interval to be 5.2 days and the incubation period as 6.5 days. There would tend to be a high presymptomatic or asymptomatic transmission of COVID-19, where the average serial interval is shorter than the average incubation period, as found in this study (Alene et al., 2021). This high viral transmissibility is further evidenced by the fact that in the USA, the first 3 million cases were hit in 167 days, from January 22, 2020, through July 8, 2020, but there were 3 million cases in the first 13 days of 2021, bringing the total number of cases to 23,067,796 and 384,604 deaths from COVID-19 during the whole pandemic (Watts & Langmaid, 2021).

SARS-CoV-2 reproduces largely in the upper and lower respiratory tract (Salzberger et al., 2020). The WHO (2020a) determined that the virus spreads through respiratory droplets and aerosols. The fatality rate of SARS was around 11%, whereas COVID-19's case fatality rate is within the range of 0.5–1.2%, indicating that COVID-19 is one-tenth as deadly as SARS (Christakis, 2020). With a higher infectivity rate and lower fatality rate than those of SARS, it becomes more problematic to control COVID-19. Higher infection and lower mortality rate, as is the case with COVID-19, infer the growing presence of a large number of infected people with the capacity to spread the disease. The notion that most of the COVID-19 cases are symptomatic is incorrect is now fully vindicated by Fauci, "What we did not know early on was that about 40–45% of the cases are asymptomatic. And recent modeling studies show that perhaps up to 50% of the transmissions occur from an asymptomatic person to an uninfected person. We cannot ignore asymptomatic infection, because that is a major component of the outbreak" (Godlee & Silberner, 2020 p. 2).

There are about 40–45% asymptomatic persons infected with SARS-CoV-2 infections (Oran & Topol, 2020), which makes it necessary to detect them to avoid the silent deep spread within the population. Oran and Topol noted that asymptomatic people can spread the virus to other people for more than 14 days, and characteristically, asymptomatic infection may be related to subclinical lung abnormalities, which can be identified. Because of the high risk for silent spread by asymptomatic persons, Oran and Topol advocated that testing programs include those without symptoms, probably until vaccinations achieve the goal of herd immunity, and so, in the interim, people should comply with the risk mitigation measures. Asymptomatic carriers are infected people who display no symptoms but are infectious and comprise about 50% of COVID-19 cases (Christakis, 2020, p. 2, Godlee & Silberner, 2020). Therefore, since depending solely on symptoms to detect cases is inadequate, testing needs to be extensive and test results returned speedily and, perhaps, immediately.

The WHO (2020b) points out that a major characteristic of an infectious disease as COVID-19 caused by SARS-CoV-2 is its severity, and fatality rates provide a sense of the severity of the disease, identify at-risk populations, and assess quality of the health care. The two fatality rates are as follows: infection fatality ratio (IFR) assesses the proportion of deaths among all infected individuals, and case fatality ratio (CFR) assesses the proportion of deaths among confirmed cases. A study (Blackburn et al., 2021) on IFR noted that since numerous (~50%) COVID-19 cases were asymptomatic, generalizable data on the correct number of people infected were deficient; therefore, mortality rates computed from confirmed cases would overestimate the infection rate as measured by the IFR; so in order to measure an accurate IFR, it is necessary to use population prevalence data from large geographic regions with reliable death data. Hence, Blackburn et al. (2021) used a statewide random sample with Indiana vital statistics data of confirmed COVID-19 deaths; they found that the overall IFR was 0.26%, and the IFR for people < age 40 was 0.01%; 60 or older 1.71%, Whites 0.18%; and non-Whites 0.59%.

Distribution of COVID-19 Deaths in the USA

Table 2.1 shows that as of July 14, 2021, Blacks were demographically overrepresented in COVID-19 deaths in Alabama, California, Colorado, Connecticut, District of Columbia (DC), Florida, Georgia, Illinois, Indiana, Kansas, Kentucky, Louisiana, Maryland, Massachusetts, Michigan, Mississippi, Missouri, Nevada, New Jersey, New York, North Carolina, Ohio, Pennsylvania, South Carolina, Tennessee, Virginia, and Wisconsin. Hispanics were demographically overrepresented in COVID-19 deaths in California, Colorado, DC, New York, Texas, and Utah. There were 10 States with the largest Black populations (Texas, Georgia, Florida, New York, North Carolina, California, Maryland, Illinois, Virginia, and Louisiana) (OMH, 2021a) and 10 States with the largest Hispanic populations (California, Texas, Florida, New York, Arizona, Illinois, New Jersey, Colorado, Georgia, and New Mexico) (OMH, 2021b).

Blacks have been demographically overrepresented in COVID-19 deaths in 9 of the 10 States with the largest Black population, and also in 18 other States and DC with smaller populations of Blacks. Hispanics have been disproportionately represented in COVID-19 deaths in 4 of the 10 States with the largest Hispanic population, and also in 1 State and DC with smaller populations of Hispanics.

The MMWR (Wortham et al., 2020) reported that from February 12, 2020 to May 18, 2020 (Table 2.2), there were about 1.3 million COVID-19 cases and 83,000

Table 2.1 COVID-19 Deaths by race/ethnicity as of July 14, 2021

Location	White % of Deaths	White % of Total Population	Black % of Deaths	Black % of Total Population	Hispanic % of Deaths	Hispanic % of Total Population
Alabama	68%	65%	30%	27%	2%	4%
Alaska	40%	60%	NA	2%	5%	7%
Arizona	52%	54%	3%	4%	31%	32%
Arkansas	78%	72%	15%	15%	4%	8%
California	32%	36%	6%	5%	48%	40%
Colorado	65%	68%	5%	4%	25%	22%
Connecticut	74%	66%	13%	10%	11%	17%
Delaware	73%	61%	22%	22%	4%	10%
District of Columbia	13%	37%	71%	45%	14%	11%
Florida	56%	53%	17%	15%	25%	27%
Georgia	58%	52%	35%	31%	6%	10%
Hawaii	9%	20%	NA	1%	7%	10%
Idaho	86%	82%	NA	1%	10%	13%
Illinois	62%	61%	18%	14%	16%	18%
Indiana	84%	79%	11%	9%	4%	7%
Iowa	92%	85%	3%	4%	3%	6%
Kansas	82%	76%	6%	5%	8%	12%
Kentucky	89%	84%	9%	8%	2%	4%
Louisiana	57%	59%	39%	32%	3%	5%
Maine	96%	93%	1%	1%	NA	2%
Maryland	50%	50%	37%	30%	9%	11%
Massachusetts	79%	70%	8%	7%	8%	12%
Michigan	71%	75%	23%	13%	4%	5%
Minnesota	86%	79%	5%	6%	3%	6%
Mississippi	56%	57%	41%	38%	1%	3%
Missouri	83%	79%	13%	11%	2%	4%
Montana	78%	86%	1%	1%	3%	4%
Nebraska	87%	79%	4%	5%	8%	11%
Nevada	51%	48%	10%	9%	25%	29%
New Hampshire	95%	90%	1%	1%	3%	4%
New Jersey	56%	54%	17%	12%	21%	21%
New Mexico	28%	37%	1%	2%	39%	49%
New York	50%	55%	21%	14%	22%	19%
North Carolina	67%	63%	26%	21%	5%	10%
North Dakota	88%	84%	1%	2%	2%	4%

Source: KFF, **2021**. KFF's State Health Facts. Data Sources: KFF analysis of Provisional Death Counts for Coronavirus Disease (COVID-**19**): Distribution of Deaths by Race and Hispanic Origin, National Center for Health Statistics. Data as of July **14, 2021**.Total State Population Distribution by Race/Ethnicity based on KFF analysis of **2019** American Community Survey. https://www.kff.org/other/state-indicator/covid-**19**-deaths-by-race-ethnicity/?currentTimeframe= 0&sortModel=%7B%22colId%22:%22Location%22,%22sort%22:%22asc%22%7D.

Table 2.1 (continued)

Location	White % of Deaths	White % of Total Population	Black % of Deaths	Black % of Total Population	Hispanic % of Deaths	Hispanic % of Total Population
Ohio	84%	79%	13%	12%	2%	4%
Oklahoma	73%	65%	7%	7%	6%	11%
Oregon	80%	75%	2%	2%	11%	13%
Pennsylvania	81%	76%	13%	10%	4%	8%
Rhode Island	84%	71%	5%	6%	8%	17%
South Carolina	64%	64%	33%	26%	2%	6%
South Dakota	86%	82%	NA	2%	1%	4%
Tennessee	78%	74%	18%	16%	3%	6%
Texas	42%	41%	11%	12%	45%	40%
Utah	73%	78%	1%	1%	16%	14%
Vermont	97%	93%	NA	1%	NA	2%
Virginia	64%	61%	25%	19%	7%	10%
Washington	71%	68%	4%	4%	12%	13%
West Virginia	96%	93%	3%	3%	0%	1%
Wisconsin	85%	81%	7%	6%	5%	7%
Wyoming	81%	84%	NA	1%	9%	10%

COVID-19-associated deaths. For this period, data on 52,166 deaths presented from 47 jurisdictions in the USA showed that the Hispanic, Black, and AI/AN populations were demographically overrepresented in COVID-19-associated deaths. For instance, Blacks had about 21% deaths, when their population was 13.4%.

The MMWR (Gold et al., 2020) reported that from May 1, 2020 to August 31, 2020, there were 114,411 COVID-19-associated deaths in 50 states and DC. For this period, the data on 114,411 deaths showed that the Hispanic and Black populations were demographically overrepresented in COVID-19-associated deaths. For instance, relating to Table 2.3, Blacks had about 19% deaths, when their population was 13.4%, and Hispanics with some 24% deaths with a population of 18.5%.

Table 2.4 again confirms that as of March 24, 2021, Hispanic, Black, and AI/AN were demographically overrepresented in COVID-19-associated deaths. For instance, Hispanics had some 38% deaths, when their population was 19.40%, Blacks with 22% deaths with a population of 12.70%, and AI/AN with about 3% deaths when their population was 0.70%.

Tables 2.2, 2.3, and 2.4 reveal the steadily increasing number of demographically overrepresented deaths among Blacks, Hispanics, and AI/AN from February 2020 through March 2021. Data show that Hispanics deaths constituted 13.8%, Blacks 21%, and AI/AN 0.3% at the end of August 2020 to Hispanics with 38% deaths, Blacks 22%, and AI/AN 3% deaths in March 2021.

Table 2.5 shows data on 13 States and DC, including the 10 States (USCB, 2001) where 60% of Blacks lived (New York, California, Texas, Florida, Georgia, Illinois,

Table 2.2 Demographic characteristics of COVID-19 deaths (February 12, 2020–May 18, 2020)

Characteristic	% deaths
Race/Ethnicity	
White	40.3
Hispanic	13.8
Black	21.0
Asian	3.9
American Indian/Alaska Native (AI/AN)	0.3
Native Hawaiian and Other Pacific Islander (NHPI)	0.1
Multiracial/Other race	2.6
Unknown	18.0
Sex	
Male	55.4
Age	
≥65	79.6

Source for data: Wortham et al. (2020)

Table 2.3 Demographic characteristics of COVID-19 deaths (May 1, 2020–August 31, 2020)

Characteristic	% deaths
Race/Ethnicity	
White	51.3
Hispanic	24.2
Black	18.7
Asian	3.5
AI/AN	1.3
NHPI/multiracial	0.5
Sex	
Male	53.3
Female	46.7
Age group	
18–29	0.5
30–39	1.4
40–49	3.5
50–64	16.4
65–74	21.7
75–84	26.0
≥85	30.4
Unknown	<0.1

Source for data: Gold et al. (2020)

Table 2.4 Age-adjusted percentages of COVID-19 deaths by race/ethnicity as of March 24, 2021

Characteristic	% deaths	Unweighted distribution of population (%)
Race/Ethnicity		
White	31.30	58.70
Hispanic	38.10	19.40
Black	22.30	12.70
Asian	3.70	5.80
AI/AN	2.70	0.70
Other	1.10	2.30
NHPI	0.70	0.20

Sources for data: NCHS and NVSS (2021)

North Carolina, Maryland, Michigan, and Louisiana), 4 States (Krogstad, 2020) where 45% of Hispanics lived (California, Texas, Arizona, and New Mexico), and 3 States (Soergel, 2019) where 31% of AI/AN lived (California, Arizona, and Oklahoma).

The disaggregation of data from Table 2.5 created Table 2.6, which shows that Blacks had a demographic overrepresentation in COVID-19 deaths in DC, Georgia, Illinois, Louisiana, Maryland, Michigan, New York, and North Carolina; Hispanics experienced overrepresentation in COVID-19 deaths in California, DC, New York, and Texas; and AI/AN had maximum COVID-19 deaths in Arizona, New Mexico, and Oklahoma.

Table 2.7 highlights the experiences of Blacks with a disproportionate share in COVID-19 deaths in selected counties in Florida and Georgia. Counties in Florida with a high demographic overrepresentation in COVID-19 deaths among Blacks included Alachua County (29% deaths, 20% of population), Clay County (19% deaths, 12% of population), and Leon County (37% deaths, 31% of population). Here is a profile of these Counties (IBRC, 2021): In Alachua County, for the population aged above 25, 21% completed high school, while 22% had a bachelor's degree; in 2019, median household income was US$ 49,880 and poverty rate was 18.4%; and average household size was 2.5. Relating to Clay County, for the population aged above 25, 31% finished high school and 17% had a bachelor's degree, median household income was US$ 75,776 with poverty rate at 8% in 2019, and average household size was 2.8. For the population above age 25 in Leon County, 19% completed high school with 26% having a bachelor's degree, median household income was at US$ 55,081 with poverty rate at 20.8% in 2019, and average household size was 2.4.

Counties in Georgia with a high demographic overrepresentation in COVID-19 deaths among Blacks included Bulloch County (45% deaths; 29% of population), Coweta County (31% deaths; 18% of population), Fayette County (49% deaths; 25% of population), Fulton County (55% deaths; 44% of population), and Upson County (38% deaths; 28% of population). Here is a profile of these counties (IBRC, 2021): In Bulloch County, for the population above age 25, 27% completed high

Table 2.5 Cases, hospitalizations, and deaths by States and DC with the largest Black and Hispanic populations, including AI/AN, as of March 7, 2021 (The Atlantic, 2021)

State: Arizona	**State: California**
Blacks: 4% of population; 4% of cases; 3% of deaths; 4% of hospitalizations	Blacks: 6% of population; 4% of cases; 6% of deaths; 6% of tests
AI/AN: 4% of population; 6% of cases; 9% of deaths	AI/AN: <1% of population; <1% of cases; <1% of deaths
Hispanic: 31% of population; 36% of cases; 31% of deaths; 33% of hospitalizations	Hispanics: 39% of population; 55% of cases; 46% of deaths; 30% of tests
District of Columbia	**State: Florida**
Blacks: 46% of population; 49% of cases; 76% of deaths	Blacks: 15% of population; 14% of cases; 16% of deaths; 20% of hospitalizations
AI/AN: <1% of population; <1% of cases; 0% of deaths	AI/AN: <1% of population; 0% of cases; 0% of deaths
Hispanics: 11% of population; 22% of cases; 12% of deaths	Hispanics: 26% of population; 37% of cases; 24% of deaths; 26% of hospitalizations
State: Georgia	**State: Illinois**
Blacks: 31% of population; 32% of cases; 34% of deaths; 40% of hospitalizations	Blacks: 14% of population; 13% of cases; 18% of deaths; 14% of tests
AI/AN: <1% of population; <1% of cases; <1% of deaths	AI/AN: <1% of population; <1% of cases; <1% of deaths
Hispanics: 10% of population; 13% of cases; 6% of deaths; 11% of hospitalization	Hispanics: 17% of population; 25% of cases; 16% of deaths; 13% of tests
State: Louisiana	**State: Maryland**
Blacks: 32% of population; 33% of cases; 39% of deaths	Blacks: 29% of population; 33% of cases; 35% of deaths
AI/AN: <1% of population; <1% of cases; <1% of deaths	AI/AN: <1% of population; 0% of cases; 0% of deaths
Hispanics: 5% of population; 3% of deaths	Hispanics: 10% of population; 19% of cases; 9% of deaths
State: Michigan	**State: New Mexico**
Blacks: 14% of population; 14% of cases; 23% of deaths	Blacks: 2% of population; 1% cases; 1% of deaths; 1% of hospitalizations
AI/AN: <1% of population; <1% of cases; <1% of deaths	AI/AN: 9% of population; 19% of cases; 29% of deaths
Hispanics: 5% of population; 7% of cases; 4% of deaths	Hispanics: 49% of population; 55% of cases; 40% of deaths; 42% of hospitalizations
State: New York	**State: North Carolina**
Blacks: 14% of population; case data not available; 23% of deaths; 29% of hospitalizations	Blacks: 21% of population; 21% of cases; 25% of deaths
AI/AN: <1%; 0% deaths	AI/AN: 1% of population; 2% of cases; 1% deaths
Hispanics: 19% of population; case data not available; 23% of deaths; 35% of hospitalizations	Hispanics: 9% of population; 21% of cases; 8% of deaths
State: Oklahoma	**State: Texas**
Blacks: 7% of population; 7% of cases; 7% of deaths	Blacks: 12% of population; 19% of cases; 10% of deaths

(continued)

Table 2.5   (continued)

AI/AN: 8% of population; 13% of cases; 10% of deaths	AI/AN: <1% of population; 0% of cases; 0% of deaths
Hispanics: 11% of population; 14% of cases; 6% of deaths	Hispanics: 39% of population; 41% of cases; 46% of deaths

Source for data: Adapted from The COVID Tracking Project at The Atlantic. https://covidtracking.com/race/dashboard, licensed under the terms of the Creative Commons Attribution License (https://creativecommons.org/licenses/by/4.0/)

Table 2.6   Demographic overrepresentation in clinical outcomes: Blacks, Hispanics, and AI/AN (The Atlantic, 2021)

Blacks—demographic overrepresentation in clinical outcomes by States and DC		Hispanics—demographic overrepresentation in clinical outcomes by States and DC		AI/AN— demographic overrepresentation in clinical outcomes by States	
DC	Cases and deaths	Arizona	Cases; hospitalizations	Arizona	Cases; deaths
Florida:	Hospitalizations	California	Cases; deaths	New Mexico	Cases; deaths
Georgia	Cases; deaths; hospitalizations	DC	Cases; deaths	North Carolina	Cases
Illinois	Deaths	Florida	Cases	Oklahoma	Cases; deaths
Louisiana	Cases; deaths	Georgia	Cases; hospitalizations		
Maryland	Cases; deaths	Illinois	Cases		
Michigan	Deaths	Maryland	Cases		
New York	Deaths; hospitalizations	Michigan	Cases		
North Carolina	Deaths	New Mexico	Cases		
Texas	Cases	New York	Deaths; hospitalizations		
		North Carolina	Cases		
		Oklahoma	Cases		
		Texas	Cases; deaths		

Source for data: Adapted from The COVID Tracking Project at The Atlantic. https://covidtracking.com/race/dashboard, licensed under the terms of the Creative Commons Attribution License (https://creativecommons.org/licenses/by/4.0/)

school, with 14% having a bachelor's degree, median household income was US$ 48,788 with poverty rate at 21.9% in 2019, and average household size was at 2.4. In Coweta County, for the population above age 25, 29% completed high school with 21% obtaining a bachelor's degree, median household income was US$ 79,232 with poverty rate at 9.0% in 2019, and average household size was at 2.7. Relating

Table 2.7 Counties in Florida and Georgia with COVID-19 deaths (January 1, 2020–April 17, 2021)

Data as of	Start date	End date	State	County name	Urban rural code	COVID-19 deaths	White—COVID-19 deaths (% of pop.)	Black—COVID-19 deaths (%of pop.)	Asian—COVID-19 deaths (% of pop.)	Hispanic—COVID-19 deaths (% of pop.)
4/21/2021	1/1/2020	4/17/2021	FL	Alachua County	3	614	0.668 (61)	0.285 (20)	Not available	0.036 (11)
4/21/2021	1/1/2020	4/17/2021	FL	Broward County	2	2740	0.343 (35)	0.331 (28)	0.022 (4)	0.299 (31)
4/21/2021	1/1/2020	4/17/2021	FL	Clay County	2	324	0.679 (72)	0.194 (12)	0.049 (3)	0.065 (10)
4/21/2021	1/1/2020	4/17/2021	FL	Escambia County	3	832	0.686 (64)	0.278 (23)	0.013 (3)	0.016 (6)
4/21/2021	1/1/2020	4/17/2021	FL	Leon County	3	563	0.593 (56)	0.371 (31)	Not available	0.027 (7)
4/21/2021	1/1/2020	4/17/2021	GA	Bulloch County	5	116	0.543 (63)	0.448 (29)	Not available	Not available
4/21/2021	1/1/2020	4/17/2021	GA	Coweta County	2	189	0.624 (71)	0.312 (18)	Not available	0.058 (7)
4/21/2021	1/1/2020	4/17/2021	GA	DeKalb County	2	691	0.33 (29)	0.576 (54)	0.043 (6)	0.042 (9)
4/21/2021	1/1/2020	4/17/2021	GA	Fayette County	2	256	0.461 (61)	0.488 (25)	Not available	Not available
4/21/2021	1/1/2020	4/17/2021	GA	Fulton County	1	1600	0.344 (40)	0.548 (44)	0.022 (8)	0.079 (7)
4/21/2021	1/1/2020	4/17/2021	GA	Glynn County	4	202	0.653 (64)	0.297 (26)	Not available	Not available
4/21/2021	1/1/2020	4/17/2021	GA	Houston County	4	221	0.57 (55)	0.385 (32)	Not available	Not available

(continued)

Table 2.7 (continued)

Data as of	Start date	End date	State	County name	Urban rural code	COVID-19 deaths	White— COVID-19 deaths (% of pop.)	Black— COVID-19 deaths (%of pop.)	Asian— COVID-19 deaths (% of pop.)	Hispanic— COVID-19 deaths (% of pop.)
4/21/2021	1/1/2020	4/17/2021	GA	Thomas County	5	185	0.562 (58)	0.405 (36)	Not available	Not available
4/21/2021	1/1/2020	4/17/2021	GA	Tift County	5	216	0.588 (55)	0.338 (30)	Not available	0.074 (12)
4/21/2021	1/1/2020	4/17/2021	GA	Upson County	5	154	0.61 (67)	0.383 (28)	Not available	Not available
4/21/2021	1/1/2020	4/17/2021	GA	Walton County	2	180	0.811 (73)	0.172 (18)	Not available	Not available
4/21/2021	1/1/2020	4/17/2021	GA	Ware County	5	176	0.722 (63)	0.267 (30)	Not available	Not available
4/21/2021	1/1/2020	4/17/2021	GA	Whitfield County	4	224	0.75 (57)	0.049 (4)	Not available	0.192 (36)

Source: CDC (2021b)

to Fayette County, for the population above age 25, 21% graduated from high school with 29% having a bachelor's degree, median household income was US$ 94,563 with poverty rate at 5.4% in 2019, and average household size was at 2.7. In relation to Fulton County, for the population above age 25, 18% graduated from high school with 31% having a bachelor's degree, median household income was US$ 79,235 with poverty rate at 13.8% in 2019, and average household size was at 2.4. And as per Upson County, for the population above age 25, 38% graduated from high school with 9% having a bachelor's degree, median household income was US$ 40,926 with poverty rate at 19.1% in 2019, and average household size was at 2.5.

Refer to Table 2.8 to absorb the unequal toll on COVID-19-associated hospitalizations exacted on Blacks and other people of color in the USA. Just over half of Blacks were hospitalized for cough, shortness of breath, and pneumonia, and about two-thirds for hypertension. Some two-thirds of Hispanics were hospitalized for cough and shortness of breath, and about more than half of them were for obesity, fever/chills, and pneumonia. About two-thirds of Asian/Pacific Islanders were hospitalized for cough, shortness of breath, and pneumonia, and some half of them were hospitalized for hypertension, fever/chills, and acute respiratory failure. Almost three-quarters of AI/AN were hospitalized for cough, fever/chills, and shortness of breath; some two-thirds were hospitalized for acute respiratory failure, and pneumonia; and about half were for hypertension and obesity.

However, there is a problem with the CDC data on hospitalization. CDC's COVID-NET hospitalization data, by race and ethnicity, was sourced from particular counties in 14 States, equivalent to about only 10% of the US population; thus the data is not national (Goldfarb, 2021). Additionally, 17 of the 24 States publicly presenting race/ethnicity data on hospitalizations on their own dashboards did not constitute part of the CDC's COVID-NET dataset. Even the HHS Hospitalization dataset is devoid of race/ethnicity data. In conclusion, variances in data completeness by race/ethnicity could result in understating the disparities (Labgold et al., 2021), and limitations to 14 States would reduce the generalizability of these findings because they are based on only 10% of the US population.

According to Table 2.9, compared to Whites, Blacks were 1.1 times more probable to become infected with the COVID-19 disease, 2.9 times more likely to be hospitalized, and 1.9 times more probable to die. In the same way, compared to Whites, Hispanics were 1.3 times more probable to contract the virus, 3.1 times more likely to be hospitalized, and 2.3 times more probable to die. Compared to Whites, both Blacks and Hispanics were similar in their susceptibility to contract this highly transmissible pathogen and to become hospitalized. But susceptibility may not be a strong predictor for contracting the virus. Mackey et al. (2020), in their systematic review, cited some statistical models (Azar et al., 2020; Golestaneh et al., 2020; Gu et al., 2020; Price-Haywood et al., 2020; Rentsch et al., 2020; Li et al., 2020a; Nayak et al., 2020) to signal that exposure and health-care access variables were more potent predictors for racial health disparities than susceptibility to contracting COVID-19.

Table 2.8 COVID-19-associated hospitalizations by race/ethnicity and illness as of March 14, 2021

| Hospitalization | | | | | | | | | $\bar{X}$ |
Race/Ethnicity	Diabetes (%)	Hypertension (%)	Obesity (%)	Cough (%)	Fever/chills (%)	Shortness of breath (%)	Acute respiratory failure (%)	Pneumonia (%)	%
White	32.5	63.5	45.4	56.8	46.5	61.1	44.4	52.3	50.3
Black	40.7	67.7	54.8	54.1	47.4	58	36.3	54.8	51.6
Hispanic/Latino	33.1	38	51.8	67.3	60	68.1	48.4	59.2	53.2
Asian Pacific Islander	40.1	53.7	33.6	65.9	57.3	66.9	54.9	63.4	49.9
American Indian/ Alaska Native	46.9	50.4	49.8	70.6	69.7	70.3	67.2	64.8	61.2
$\bar{X}$	38.66	47.06	47.08	51.14	56.18	64.88	50.24	58.9	

Source for data: Adapted from CDC (2021a)

Table 2.9 Risk for COVID-19 infection, hospitalization, and death by race/ethnicity

Rate ratios compared to White, Non-Hispanic persons	American Indian or Alaska Native, Non-Hispanic persons	Asian, Non-Hispanic persons	Black or African American, Non-Hispanic persons	Hispanic or Latino persons
Cases[1]	1.7x	0.7x	1.1x	1.3x
Hospitalization[2]	3.7x	1.0x	2.9x	3.1x
Death[3]	2.4x	1.0x	1.9x	2.3x

Source for data: CDC (2021c)

The effective rollout of vaccinations from January 2021 by the Biden Administration, enabling about a third of Americans to be fully vaccinated toward the end of April 2021, has certainly influenced a slow downward trend in the incidence, hospitalizations, and deaths of Americans. Nevertheless, the USA on May 24, 2021, with 33,134,618 cases and 590,141 deaths (JHU, 2021), certainly presents a tragic profile rooted in the perpetual mismanagement of the COVID-19 pandemic by the Trump Administration throughout the year 2020.

Mismanagement of the COVID-19 Pandemic

It is noteworthy that the Centers for Disease Control and Prevention (CDC) has been administering the Global Health Protection Program since its inception during the Ebola outbreak in 2014, as a result of West Africa advocacy. The Global Health Protection Program included 50 countries, inclusive of China, as a training program for disease detectives, who are vital to countries' capabilities to rapidly discover and end disease outbreaks globally. The US Congress then approved about US\$ 600 million for the CDC to support the Global Health Protection Program, in order to upscale its capacity globally to identify and suppress new infectious diseases. However, in January 2018, the head of the CDC's Center for Global Health informed the staff that the Global Health Protection Program was scaled down to only 10 countries, excluding China. The funds initially apportioned for the program were no longer available in 2019, the outcome of which was that there was no US staffer at the CDC office in Beijing at the time of the COVID-19 outbreak (Greenberg, 2020).

Over the last 10 months of the COVID-19 pandemic, largely coinciding with President Trump's last 10 months or so in the office, his Administration's incapacity to produce a preparedness and response plan, his reluctance to support adequate containment activities, and zero early interventions, has contributed to the contagion's current devastating and tragic impact on the US health-care system, with demographic disproportionate outcomes on communities of color. Three prestigious public health journals, *Scientific American*, *The Lancet*, and the *New England Journal of Medicine* (NEJM), have all published serious criticisms of the Trump Administration's mishandling of the pandemic. Referring to the COVID-19 pandemic, the NEJM (2020, pp. 1479–1480) asserted that the Trump Administration had "taken a crisis and turned it into a tragedy" and surmised the COVID-19 catastrophic impact on the American nation as:

> The magnitude of this failure is astonishing... the United States leads the world in Covid-19 cases and in deaths due to the disease, far exceeding the numbers in much larger countries, such as China. The death rate in this country is more than double that of Canada, exceeds that of Japan, a country with a vulnerable and elderly population, by a factor of almost 50, and even dwarfs the rates in lower-middle-income countries, such as Vietnam, by a factor of almost 2000.

The NEJM found that US testing was ineffective; was well below the curve in testing as it failed to meet the standards on the number of tests administered per infected person, with long delays in issuing test results; and was unable to deliver basic personal protective equipment (PPE) to health-care workers. The NEJM editors further noted that quarantine and isolation prevention measures were introduced late and inconsistently, with minimum enforcement, as the community spread of the disease gained momentum. The NEJM editors also noted that social distancing was apathetic, where restrictions were relaxed well before there was any control of the disease and many people did not wear masks as leaders saw them as political tools rather than as primary infection control measures.

The Trump Administration's mismanagement of the COVID-19 pandemic has brought untold damage to Blacks and other communities of color. Given invariably their context of poverty and limited and/or no health care, it is not surprising that each time the USA faces a public health crisis of the magnitude of the COVID-19 pandemic, Blacks, particularly and indisputably, become the most victimized casualties of huge racial health disparities and structural disadvantage. Such perpetual and tragic existential crisis repeatedly prompts many to throw their hands in the air looking for genuine answers, which are ubiquitous for those sincerely interested in improving and equalizing health outcomes for all in American society. Clearly, instead of COVID-19 being an equalizer, given its capacity to infect all and sundry, Blacks have been demographically overrepresented in the areas of COVID-19 cases, hospitalizations, and deaths.

Then there has been the issue of inadequate compilation of data on people of color. But the growing problem of incomplete data on race and ethnicity for one-third of COVID-19 cases impairs actions to mitigate COVID-19 racial health disparities (Krieger et al., 2020). In addition, since race and ethnicity have been missing from data on cases, it is possible that counties with considerable missing data may be omitted for any analysis on racial health disparities; as a remedy to this difficulty posed by case-based analysis, population-based studies could be utilized to focus interventions (Lee et al., 2021); and over the period of April 1–14, 2020, 11.4% of counties, mainly in the Northeast and South, presented high COVID-19 incidence, comprising 28.7% of the counties with a huge Asian population and 27.9% of the counties with a sizeable Black population. Lee et al. (2021) noted that within the

August 5–18, 2020, period, it increased to 64.7% of counties, largely in the South, with 92.4% of the counties having a large Black population and 74.5% of the counties carrying a substantial Hispanic population; then around December 9–22, 2020, when 99.1% of the counties presented high COVID-19 incidence, >95% of the counties with considerable populations of each racial and ethnic minority group accounted for high COVID-19 incidence.

Early in the pandemic, testing was delayed because of Trump's unending denial of the pathogen's presence, and the Trump Administration's subtle reluctance to utilize the WHO test kit, but only to discover that its own test kit was deficient. *Science* (Cohen, 2020) reported that in the early days of the pandemic, the WHO had already sent testing kits to 57 countries. China by that time was administering five commercial tests with a capacity to conduct up to 1.6 million tests weekly and South Korea had tested 65,000 persons. However, in comparison, the CDC administered only 459 tests from the commencement of the epidemic to circa February 2020, and to compound the CDC's problems, the rollout of its test kit to state and local laboratories was a mess, as it had a faulty reagent. Coupled with this bungling in the commencement of testing was the massive shortage of basic PPE for health-care workers and the public.

The COVID-19 testing disaster was predictable with former President Trump perpetually in denial on the emergence of the virus, as evidenced by some of his comments and his Administration's response (Doggett, 2021). The USA clearly started testing for COVID-19 later than many countries, contrary to President Trump's assertions. *Our World in Data* (GCDL, 2021) provided the following information: On April 15, 2020, the USA tested 3,120,381 people from a total population of 328 million. On April 13, 2020, the USA did 8.86 tests per 1000 people; on April 5, 2020, Germany did 15.97 tests per 1000 people; on April 14, 2020, Ireland did 18.55 tests per 1000 people; on April 13, 2020, Israel did 19.75 tests per 1000 people; on April 14, 2020, Canada did 11.63 tests per 1000 people; and on April 13, 2020, New Zealand did 13.32 tests per 1000 people.

Howard Forman, Director of Yale School of Public Health (Snouwaert, 2020), in early 2020 advised on the need for COVID-19 tests to instill confidence that the virus was contained. He argued then for broad-scale testing, a critical step, to adequately contain and mitigate the spread of COVID-19. But especially in the early months of the pandemic, the US testing was inadequate, which might have resulted in cases exploding in the near future. He explained further that the increase in undetected cases may have induced the spread of COVID-19. At that time, this low level of testing as per the size of the pandemic suggested that a true number of infections in the USA was probably greater than the number of confirmed cases. The number of infected might have been even larger because only those with the most severe symptoms were being tested. Those with mild symptoms or no symptoms were not tested; thus, chances were that the infected number was larger than what was presented. In addition, the USA had no national testing program, and so, the burden of testing fell on States and private businesses.

The COVID-19 testing debacle and the absence of a preparedness plan compounded the US response in the early months of this pandemic. Then on June 22,

2021, a study (Kalish et al., 2021) noted that asymptomatic SARS-CoV-2 infection and late implementation of diagnostics resulted in poorly defined viral prevalence rates in the USA and found that there were 4.8 undiagnosed SARS-CoV-2 infections for every diagnosed case of COVID-19, with an estimated 16.8 million undiagnosed infections by mid-July 2020 in the USA. Besides, in an interview with the British Medical Journal, Fauci emphasized the significance of asymptomatic people in this pandemic (Godlee & Silberner, 2020).

Amid the growing COVID-19 pandemic during 2020, former President Trump mismanaged the pandemic not only through his constant denial of the existential threat of the contagion but also through his announcement of severing the US link with the WHO, no preparedness and response plan, limited health literacy for understanding the rationale for containment and mitigation measures, the reluctance to increase testing, his divisive strategy of advantaging purported "Republican" States, and disavowing soi-disant "Democratic" States. This bungling approach to COVID-19 totally disrupted field epidemiology "with the goal of immediate action to address a public health problem of concern" (Goodman et al., 2019). How so?

Field epidemiology requires diagnostic testing. Delays in testing were a constant public health response, which contributed to the vagueness of the disease burden as well as the scope of the spread. After the first case in the USA was detected on January 21, 2020, there was an acceleration of the contagion between February and March 2020 vis-à-vis constant travel-associated imports, huge gatherings, high-risk workplaces and densely populated areas, and a cryptic spread following limited testing and asymptomatic and presymptomatic spread. These missteps compromised public health interventions necessary to reduce the community spread (Schuchat & Team, 2020).

Field epidemiology suggests that we identify the social determinants of health early to accelerate interventions to reduce such atrocities against people of color. But these are the same racial/ethnic groups that constantly experience disproportionality in clinical outcomes time and again. Thus, the demographic overrepresentation in cases, hospitalizations, and deaths amid COVID-19 should not be surprising, as even the *Healthy People 2020* (ODPHP, 2020) approach to the social determinants of health does not prominently include systemic racism as one of the determinants.

Authentic primary communications within the COVID-19 pandemic are critical, and yet during 2020, politicians and not public health experts were largely the messengers (Gollust et al., 2020), which is a breach of field epidemiology guidance. Messaging should also improve public health literacy issues, as educating people to understand the rationale for interventions (wear masks, maintain physical distance, wash hands, get vaccinated, etc.) to reduce community spread.

Targeted evidence-based interventions should be implemented early to reduce community spread, which is a core significance of field epidemiology. For instance, evidence from the European Centre for Disease Prevention and Control on policies implemented in 149 countries found that physical distancing interventions at school and workplace, closures, limitations on huge gatherings, lockdowns, etc. reduced incidence of COVID-19. Over a year of the pandemic, large numbers of people in the USA were experiencing COVID-19 fatigue, and there were some sections of the population who were politically motivated to disregard the primary prevention measures.

The mismanagement of the vaccine distribution compounded the problem. For instance, with approval for emergency use authorization (EUA) of two vaccines, Pfizer-BioNTech, and Moderna in late 2020 in the USA, federal government officials estimated that 20 million Americans would be vaccinated by December 31, 2020; the CDC showed that about 11.4 million doses were distributed as of December 28, 2020, but only about 2.1 million were administered, well short of Operation Warp Speed's initial goal of 20 million inoculations by December 31, 2020 (Kaufman et al., 2020). Thus, with limited vaccine distribution, a situation that won't be ameliorated until early 2021, usage of limited therapeutics, and the perpetual high viral transmissibility, complying with preventive measures such as social distancing and wearing masks, becomes absolutely necessary to contain the community spread of the contagion.

Within this pandemic, field epidemiology supports the sustainability of global partnerships for countries to work together against any global health threat. But on May 29, 2020, former President Trump announced his intention to sever the US link with the WHO (D. G. Mcneil & Jacobs, 2020). Indeed, President Joe Biden has now reversed any delinking. Through the International Health Regulations 2005 framework, the WHO issued the strategic preparedness and response plan in 2020 to coordinate global action against COVID-19, and recently the WHO issued the 2021 version. Interestingly, during 2020, the USA had no plan to combat the pandemic (Tanne, 2020), especially given its high transmissibility, which is one of its formidable epidemiologic characteristics. Undoubtedly, the high infectivity of COVID-19, like other disease outbreaks and epidemics, has once more exposed racial health disparities, powered by systemic racism, bringing unspeakable damage to Blacks and other racially disadvantaged communities of color.

References

Alene, M., Yismaw, L., Assemie, M. A., Ketema, D. B., Gietaneh, W., & Birhan, T. Y. (2021). Serial interval and incubation period of COVID-19: A systematic review and meta-analysis. *BMC Infectious Diseases, 21*, 257.

Azar, K. M., Shen, Z., Romanelli, R. J., Lockhart, S. H., Smits, K., Robinson, S., Brown, S., & Pressman, A. R. (2020). Disparities in outcomes among COVID-19 patients in A large health care system in California: Study estimates the COVID-19 infection fatality rate at the US county level. *Health Affairs, 39*, 1253–1262.

Blackburn, J., Yiannoutsos, C. T., Carroll, A. E., Halverson, P. K., & Menachemi, N. (2021). Infection fatality ratios for COVID-19 among noninstitutionalized persons 12 and older: Results of a random-sample prevalence study. *Annals of Internal Medicine, 174*, 135–136.

CDC. (2021a). *Characteristics of COVID-19-associated hospitalizations from the COVID-NET network (data downloaded on 3/14/2021)* [Online]. CDC. Available: https://gis.cdc.gov/grasp/COVIDNet/COVID19_5.html. Accessed 14 Mar 2021.

CDC. (2021b). *Provisional COVID-19 death counts by county and race* [Online]. CDC. Available: https://data.cdc.gov/NCHS/Provisional-COVID-19-Death-Counts-by-County-and-Ra/k8wy-p9cg/data. Accessed 14 Apr 2021.

CDC. (2021c). *Risk for COVID-19 infection, hospitalization, and death by race/ethnicity* [Online]. CDC. Available: https://www.cdc.gov/coronavirus/2019-ncov/covid-data/investigations-discovery/hospitalization-death-by-race-ethnicity.html. Accessed 18 Mar 2021.

Christakis, N. (2020). Fighting covid-19 by truly understanding the virus. *The Economist, 10.*

Cohen, J. (2020). *The United States badly bungled coronavirus testing—But things may soon improve* [Online]. Science, AAAS. Available: https://www.sciencemag.org/news/2020/02/united-states-badly-bungled-coronavirus-testing-things-may-soon-improve.   Accessed   19 May 2021.

Doggett, L. (2021). *Timeline of Trump's coronavirus responses* [online]. U.S. House of Representatives. Available: https://doggett.house.gov/media-center/blog-posts/timeline-trumps-coronavirus-responses. Accessed 25 June 2021.

Du, Z., Xu, X., Wu, Y., Wang, L., Cowling, B. J., & Meyers, L. A. (2020). Serial interval of COVID-19 among publicly reported confirmed cases. *Emerging Infectious Diseases, 26,* 1341.

GCDL. (2021). *Coronavirus pandemic (COVID-19)* [online]. Oxford Martin School, University of Oxford, GCDL. Available: https://ourworldindata.org/coronavirus. Accessed 28 Apr 2021.

Godlee, F., & Silberner, J. (2020). The BMJ interview: Anthony Fauci on covid-19. *BMJ, 370,* m3703.

Gold, Jeremy AW, Lauren M. Rossen, Farida B. Ahmad, Paul Sutton, Zeyu Li, Phillip P. Salvatore, Jayme P. Coyle et al. (2020). *Race, ethnicity, and age trends in persons who died from COVID-19 — United States, May–August 2020* [online]. MMWR, CDC. Available: https://doi.org/10.15585/mmwr.mm6942e1. Accessed 25 Mar 2021.

Goldfarb, A. (2021). *Federal COVID data 101: What we know about race and ethnicity data* [online]. The Atlantic. Available: https://covidtracking.com/analysis-updates/federal-covid-data-101-race-ethnicity-data. Accessed 23 Mar 2021.

Golestaneh, L., Neugarten, J., Fisher, M., Billett, H. H., Gil, M. R., Johns, T., Yunes, M., Mokrzycki, M. H., Coco, M., & Norris, K. C. (2020). The association of race and COVID-19 mortality. *EClinicalMedicine, 25,* 100455.

Gollust, S. E., Nagler, R. H., & Fowler, E. F. (2020). The emergence of COVID-19 in the US: A public health and political communication crisis. *Journal of Health Politics, Policy and Law, 45,* 967–981.

Goodman, R. A., Buehler, J. W., Mott, J. A., Goodman, R., Buehler, J., & Mott, J. (2019). *Defining field epidemiology*. Oxford University Press.

Greenberg, J. (2020). *Under Donald Trump, key CDC US staff in China fell to 0* [Online]. Available: https://www.politifact.com/factchecks/2020/may/21/joe-biden/under-donald-trump-key-cdc-us-staff-china-fell-0/. Accessed 5 Jan 2021.

Gu, T., Mack, J. A., Salvatore, M., Sankar, S. P., Valley, T. S., Singh, K., Nallamothu, B. K., Kheterpal, S., Lisabeth, L., & Fritsche, L. G. (2020). Characteristics associated with racial/ethnic disparities in COVID-19 outcomes in an academic health care system. *JAMA Network Open, 3,* e2025197.

Hao, X., Cheng, S., Wu, D., Wu, T., Lin, X., & Wang, C. (2020). Reconstruction of the full transmission dynamics of COVID-19 in Wuhan. *Nature, 584,* 420–424.

IBRC. (2021). *USA counties in profile* [online]. Indiana University, IN: IBRC, Indiana University. Available: https://www.statsamerica.org/USCP/#. Accessed 12 May 2021.

ICTV. (2020). The species severe acute respiratory syndrome-related coronavirus: Classifying 2019-nCoV and naming it SARS-CoV-2. *Nature Microbiology, 5,* 536.

Inglesby, T. V. (2020). Public health measures and the reproduction number of SARS-CoV-2. *JAMA.*

JHU. (2021). *COVID-19 data in motion: Monday, may 24, 2021* [online]. JHUCRC. Available: https://coronavirus.jhu.edu/. Accessed 24 May 2021.

Kalish, H., Klumpp-Thomas, C., Hunsberger, S., Baus, H. A., Fay, M. P., Siripong, N., Wang, J., Hicks, J., Mehalko, J., Travers, J., Drew, M., Pauly, K., Spathies, J., Ngo, T., Adusei, K. M.,

Karkanitsa, M., Croker, J. A., Li, Y., Graubard, B. I., … Sadtler, K. (2021). Undiagnosed SARS-CoV-2 seropositivity during the first six months of the COVID-19 pandemic in the United States. *Science Translational Medicine*, eabh3826.

Kaufman, E., Grayer, A., Murray, S. & Kane, A. (2020). *US officials promised 20 million vaccinated against coronavirus by the end of the year. It's going slower than that* [Online]. Available: https://www.cnn.com/2020/12/23/health/vaccine-rollout-slow-data-lags/index.html. Accessed 14 Jan 2021.

KFF. (2021). *COVID-19 Deaths by Race/Ethnicity. Timeframe as of July 14, 2021. State Health Facts* [Online]. Available: https://www.kff.org/other/state-indicator/covid-19-deaths-by-race-ethnicity/?currentTimeframe=0&sortModel=%7B%22colId%22:%22Location%22,%22sort%22:%22asc%22%7D. Accessed 14 July 2021.

Krieger, N., Testa, C., Hanage, W. P., & Chen, J. T. (2020). US racial and ethnic data for COVID-19 cases: Still missing in action. *The Lancet, 396*, e81.

Krogstad, J. M. (2020). *Hispanics have accounted for more than half of total U.S. population growth since 2010* [Online]. Pew Research Center. Available: https://www.pewresearch.org/fact-tank/2020/07/10/hispanics-have-accounted-for-more-than-half-of-total-u-s-population-growth-since-2010/. Accessed 1 Apr 2021.

Labgold, K., Hamid, S., Shah, S., Gandhi, N. R., Chamberlain, A., Khan, F., Khan, S., Smith, S., Williams, S., & Lash, T. L. (2021). Estimating the unknown: Greater racial and ethnic disparities in COVID-19 burden after accounting for missing race and ethnicity data. *Epidemiology, 32*, 157–161.

Lee, F. C., Adams, L., Graves, S. J., Massetti, G. M., & Calanan, R. M. (2021). *Counties with high COVID-19 incidence and relatively large racial and ethnic minority populations — United States, April 1–December 22, 2020* [online]. MMWR, CDC. Available: https://www.cdc.gov/mmwr/volumes/70/wr/pdfs/mm7013e1-H.pdf. Accessed 26 Mar 2021.

Li, A. Y., Hannah, T. C., Durbin, J. R., Dreher, N., Mcauley, F. M., Marayati, N. F., Spiera, Z., Ali, M., Gometz, A., & Kostman, J. (2020a). Multivariate analysis of black race and environmental temperature on COVID-19 in the US. *The American Journal of the Medical Sciences, 360*, 348–356.

Li, Q., Guan, X., Wu, P., Wang, X., Zhou, L., Tong, Y., Ren, R., Leung, K. S., Lau, E. H., & Wong, J. Y. (2020b). Early transmission dynamics in Wuhan, China, of novel coronavirus–infected pneumonia. *New England Journal of Medicine*.

Li, Q., Guan, X., Wu, P., Wang, X., Zhou, L., Tong, Y., Ren, R., Leung, K. S. M., Lau, E. H. Y., Wong, J. Y., Xing, X., Xiang, N., Wu, Y., Li, C., Chen, Q., Li, D., Liu, T., Zhao, J., Liu, M., … Feng, Z. (2020c). Early transmission dynamics in Wuhan, China, of novel coronavirus-infected pneumonia. *The New England Journal of Medicine, 382*, 1199–1207.

Liu, Q., Xu, K., Wang, X., & Wang, W. (2020). From SARS to COVID-19: What lessons have we learned? *Journal of Infection and Public Health, 13*, 1611–1618.

Mackey, K., Ayers, C. K., Kondo, K. K., Saha, S., Advani, S. M., Young, S., Spencer, H., Rusek, M., Anderson, J., Veazie, S., Smith, M., & Kansagara, D. (2020). Racial and ethnic disparities in COVID-19-related infections, hospitalizations, and deaths: A systematic review. *Annals of Internal Medicine*.

Mcneil, D. G., & Jacobs, A. (2020). Blaming China for pandemic, trump says U.S. will leave the W.H.O. [online]. *The New York times*. Available: https://www.nytimes.com/2020/05/29/health/virus-who.html. Accessed 21 Mar 2021.

Nayak, A., Islam, S. J., Mehta, A., Ko, Y.-A., Patel, S. A., Goyal, A., Sullivan, S., Lewis, T. T., Vaccarino, V. & Morris, A. A. (2020). Impact of social vulnerability on COVID-19 incidence and outcomes in the United States. *medRxiv*.

NCHS & NVSS. (2021). *Health disparities: Race and Hispanic origin* [online]. NCHS/NVSS, CDC. Available: https://www.cdc.gov/nchs/nvss/vsrr/covid19/health_disparities.htm. Accessed 25 Mar 2021.

NEJM. (2020). Dying in a leadership vacuum. *New England Journal of Medicine, 383*, 1479–1480.

Nishiura, H., Linton, N. M., & Akhmetzhanov, A. R. (2020). Serial interval of novel coronavirus (COVID-19) infections. *International Journal of Infectious Diseases*.

ODPHP. (2020). *Social determinants of health* [Online]. U.S. Department of Health and Human Services. Available: https://www.healthypeople.gov/2020/topics-objectives/topic/social-determinants-of-health. Accessed 27 Apr 2021.

Olney, A. M., Smith, J., Sen, S., Thomas, F., & Unwin, H. J. T. (2020). Estimating the effect of social distancing interventions on COVID-19 in the United States. *medRxiv*.

OMH. (2021a). *Profile: Black/African Americans* [online]. U.S. Department of Health and Human Services, OMH. Available: https://www.minorityhealth.hhs.gov/omh/browse.aspx?lvl=3&lvlid=61. Accessed 5 May 2021.

OMH. (2021b). *Profile: Hispanic/Latino Americans* [Online]. U.S. Department of Health and Human Services, OMH. Available: https://minorityhealth.hhs.gov/omh/browse.aspx?lvl=3&lvlid=64. Accessed 5 May 2021.

Oran, D. P., & Topol, E. J. (2020). Prevalence of asymptomatic SARS-CoV-2 infection: A narrative review. *Annals of Internal Medicine, 173*, 362–367.

Park, S. E. (2020). Epidemiology, virology, and clinical features of severe acute respiratory syndrome -coronavirus-2 (SARS-CoV-2; coronavirus Disease-19). *Clinical and Experimental Pediatrics, 63*, 119–124.

Park, M., Cook, A. R., Lim, J. T., Sun, Y., & Dickens, B. L. (2020). A systematic review of COVID-19 epidemiology based on current evidence. *Journal of Clinical Medicine, 9*, 967.

Price-Haywood, E. G., Burton, J., Fort, D., & Seoane, L. (2020). Hospitalization and mortality among black patients and white patients with Covid-19. *New England Journal of Medicine, 382*, 2534–2543.

Rentsch, C. T., Kidwai-Khan, F., Tate, J. P., Park, L. S., King, J. T., Jr., Skanderson, M., Hauser, R. G., Schultze, A., Jarvis, C. I., & Holodniy, M. (2020). Covid-19 by race and ethnicity: A national cohort study of 6 million United States veterans. *MedRxiv*.

Sandman, P. M. (2007). *A severe pandemic is not overdue - it's not when but if* [Online]. University of Minnesota: CIDRAP - Center for Infectious Disease Research and Policy. Available: https://www.cidrap.umn.edu/news-perspective/2007/02/severepandemic-not-overdue-its-not-when-if [Accessed October 26, 2021].

Salzberger, B., Buder, F., Lampl, B., Ehrenstein, B., Hitzenbichler, F., Holzmann, T., Schmidt, B., & Hanses, F. (2020). Epidemiology of SARS-CoV-2. *Infection*, 1–7.

Schuchat, A., & Team, C. C.-R. (2020). Public health response to the initiation and spread of pandemic COVID-19 in the United States, February 24-April 21, 2020. *MMWR. Morbidity and Mortality Weekly Report, 69*, 551–556.

Snouwaert, J. (2020). *'We are in a crisis here': The Yale professor who said US coronavirus cases were set to 'explode' in the coming days warns that America is way behind on testing* [Online]. Business Insider. Available: https://www.businessinsider.com/coronavirus-covid-19-tests-needed-united-states-crisis-yale-professor-2020-3. Accessed 28 Apr 2021.

Soergel, A. (2019). *Where Most native Americans live* [online]. U.S. News & World Report. Available: https://www.usnews.com/news/best-states/articles/2019-11-29/california-arizona-oklahoma-where-most-native-americans-live. Accessed 1 Apr 2021.

Tanne, J. H. (2020). Covid-19: US needs a national plan to fight rising infections, experts say. *BMJ, 370*, m3072.

The Atlantic. (2021). *Racial data dashboard* [online]. The COVID Tracking Project, The Atlantic. Available: https://covidtracking.com/race/dashboard. Accessed 18 Mar 2021.

USCB. (2001). *Majority of African Americans live in 10 states; new York City and Chicago are cities with largest black populations* [Online]. U.S. Department of Commerce. Available: https://www.census.gov/newsroom/releases/archives/census_2000/cb01cn176.html. Accessed 1 Apr 2021.

Watts, A. & Langmaid, V. (2021). *3 million new US Covid-19 cases were diagnosed in the past 13 days* [Online]. Available: https://www.cnn.com/world/live-news/coronavirus-pandemic-vaccine-updates-01-13-21/index.html. Accessed 14 Jan 2021.

WHO (2020a). *Report of the WHO-China joint mission on coronavirus disease 2019 (COVID-19)*.

WHO. (2020b). *Scientific brief* [online]. WHO. Available: https://www.who.int/news-room/com-mentaries/detail/estimating-mortality-from-covid-19. Accessed 10 Aug 2021.

WHO. (2020c). *WHO director-General's opening remarks at the media briefing on COVID-19 – 11 march 2020* [online]. WHO. Available: https://www.who.int/director-general/speeches/detail/who-director-general-s-opening-remarks-at-the-media-briefing-on-covid-19%2D%2D-11-march-2020. Accessed 26 Apr 2021.

WMHC. (2020). *Press statement related to novel coronavirus infection (in Chinese)* [Online]. Available: http://wjw.wuhan.gov.cn/front/web/showDetail/2020012709194. Accessed 18 Jan 2021.

Wortham, J. M., Lee, J. T., Althomsons, S., Latash, J., Davidson, A., Guerra, K. & Murray, K. (2020). *Characteristics of persons who died with COVID-19 — United States, February 12–May 18, 2020* [online]. MMWR, CDC. Available: https://doi.org/10.15585/mmwr.mm6928e1externali-con. Accessed 25 Mar 2021.

Xiang, Y., Jia, Y., Chen, L., Guo, L., Shu, B., & Long, E. (2021). COVID-19 epidemic predic-tion and the impact of public health interventions: A review of COVID-19 epidemic models. *Infectious Disease Modelling, 6*, 324–342.

Zhou, P., Yang, X.-L., Wang, X.-G., Hu, B., Zhang, L., Zhang, W., Si, H.-R., Zhu, Y., Li, B., & Huang, C.-L. (2020). A pneumonia outbreak associated with a new coronavirus of probable bat origin. *Nature, 579*, 270–273.

Chapter 3
Systemic Racism and the White Racial Frame

A Historical Overview

The White racial frame (Feagin, 2020), through its permeation of every fabric of society, controls the health system. After 402 years, the Black health crisis, racial health disparities, with health inequalities and health inequities, and the segregated health system, have remained an existential reality. These realities are deeply embedded in a culture of persisting and growing racism, even now as America is being ravaged by a raging and highly transmissible contagion, COVID-19. This pandemic has exposed troubling racial health disparities and inequities in its demographically disproportionate impact on Blacks and other people of color. The reasons generally proffered for the disparities relate to the Black body or inequalities that shaped Black history (Hammonds & Reverby, 2019), but many studies of racial health disparities have ignored the history of the Black experience (Chowkwanyun, 2011).

To be clear, reinstatement of a state-of-the-art historical analysis adds flavor and strength to an interdisciplinary approach to public health. A historical perspective offers a sense of the reasons in the past for this persisting racial health disparities, relating them to the body and the body politic, enabling public health practitioners to disable the burdens impacting Blacks' conditions of living (Hammonds & Reverby, 2019). The historical outlook shows that "White-imposed racism" with racial oppression, manifested through slavery and legal segregation, was part of the structural foundation of the USA (Feagin, 2020), as well as through genocide and dispossession of the Indigenous people through settler colonialism (McKay et al., 2020). Settler colonialism (McKay et al., 2020) portrayed the genocide and dispossession of the Indigenous people, depicted the White colonizers' settlement on lands already owned and occupied by the Indigenous people, and delivered the framework, where White supremacy has flourished through the construction, execution, and sustainability of race and racism; thus, the White colonizers' land theft,

P. Misir, *COVID-19 and Health System Segregation in the US*, Springer Briefs in Public Health, https://doi.org/10.1007/978-3-030-88766-7_3

commodification, selling, and management of Indigenous lands were fundamental to the beginnings of White-imposed racism in the USA.

One of the consequences of slavery was the establishment of racially segregated health care, where slave owners perceived Black bodies as requiring discipline and control, in order to keep them fit for labor. While on the other hand, the enslaved Africans utilized skills acquired from their homelands in Africa and used roots, herbs, and communal support to tend to the sick among them (Hammonds & Reverby, 2019). Aside from some sporadic instances of legal progression to wipe out racial oppression, White-imposed racism remains a penetrative force embedded in the American life currently and, specifically, too, as a fundamental cause of racial health disparities (Phelan & Link, 2015; Boyd et al., 2020; Yearby, 2020; Hardeman, 2020; Garcia et al., 2020; Mccord & Freeman, 1990; Ogedegbe, 2020; Beck et al., 2020; Pirtle, 2020; Williams et al., 2019; Serchen et al., 2020).

Around the turn of the century, Du Bois in "The Forethought" to his book, *The Souls of Black Folk* (Du Bois, 2008), mentioned the strange meaning of being Black, expressing his concerns about Black lives and the aftermath of the Black enslavement. He firmly upheld the view that the problem of the twentieth century would become the problem of the color line. At that time, the Black population was 9,204,531 (Wilcox, 1904). In *The Souls of Black Folk* (Du Bois, 2008 p. 5), Du Bois vehemently voiced the persisting double consciousness Blacks faced and the devastating impact of Black enslavement:

> …the Negro is a sort of seventh son, born with a veil, and gifted with second-sight in this American world, —a world which yields him no true self-consciousness, but only lets him see himself through the revelation of the other world…this double-consciousness…One ever feels his twoness, – an American, a Negro; two souls, two thoughts, two unreconciled strivings; two warring ideals in one dark body….

It is now well established that the American society's foundational reality was extreme racial oppression, rooted and shaped by Indigenous genocide and dispossession, Black enslavement, and legal racial segregation along the color line. Du Bois' problem of the color line (Du Bois, 2008), a defining and fundamental problem of race in the twentieth century, has extended its dominance into the twenty-first century, with intensified institutional practices of racism and White supremacy gaining momentum. The color line, as Du Bois (2008) signaled, prevents Blacks from developing true self-consciousness, resulting in their subordination to and domination by "Whiteness" (Du Bois, 1920), which had become a new religion in society, molded by this color line and racial hierarchies created by the dominant Whites.

Du Bois' concept of the color line, perhaps, also impacting the other people of color faced with similar attendant problems of double consciousness and marginalization as Blacks, emerges now with a new narrative to sustain and drive its domination through a new slogan "…of egalitarian hopes and post-racial rhetoric of the recent American experience…" (Bobo, 2017). Notwithstanding that for centuries, Blacks' unrelenting yearning for freedom has remained elusive, so any end to dominance and control would require a logic of targeted action to obliterate the White-imposed racism in the current times. About 250 years ago, the White colonists in

America secured their freedom from the British with a similar logic of directed action, demanding an end to imperial dominance and control. That logic defined the battle cry for the birth of a free United States of America in 1776, founded on the principle of the *Declaration of Independence* (Jefferson, 1776):

> ...We hold these truths to be self-evident, that all men are created equal, that they are endowed by their Creator with certain unalienable Rights, that among these are Life, Liberty and the pursuit of Happiness....

This principle is extensively observed as representing the genesis of a novel and unique American history, focused on advancing a progressive development of rights (Ostler, 2020), and signaling the founding of a new era of progressive governance and a new America. But it is noteworthy and not surprising to recognize that the 1776 *Declaration of Independence*, principally authored by prominent slaveholder Thomas Jefferson, was denied to slaves, and in the final draft, Jefferson deleted the clause condemning slavery, a position quite consistent with the final clause of this Declaration (Jefferson, 1776). The Declaration itself, essentially, comprised grievances against King George III, thus:

> He has excited domestic insurrections amongst us, and has endeavoured to bring on the inhabitants of our frontiers, the merciless Indian Savages, whose known rule of warfare, is an undistinguished destruction of all ages, sexes and conditions.

The Declaration's closing statement delivered two hard truths about America's founding that, invariably, have been ignored. For those White colonists who pursued independence in 1776, the first hard truth was designed at preserving the institution of slavery (Ostler, 2020). They accomplished this feat by castigating King George III for inciting slave revolts, aimed at ending 250 years of slavery. Within this context, it is significant to explain the reason for acknowledging "250 years and not 157 years of servitude." It is important to recognize that the first enslaved Africans landed in the USA not in 1619 as is widely acknowledged, but in 1526, when a Spanish expedition with enslaved Africans created a settlement in South Carolina, and in November of 1526, the enslaved Africans rebelled and demolished the Spanish settlers' capacity to maintain the settlement (Guasco, 2017). Thus, at the time of the 1776 *Declaration of Independence*, enslaved Africans already were in the USA for 250 years.

The second hard truth (Ostler, 2020) was aimed at suppressing Native American resistance vis-à-vis accusing George III for unleashing "the merciless Indian Savages" upon "inhabitants of our frontiers." Ostler, nevertheless, contended that the increased Native American violence was provoked by White colonists' invasion of Native lands west of the Appalachian Mountains. The upshot was the banding together of the Senecas, Shawnees, Delawares, Ottawas, Cherokees, and other Native nations, using their right of self-defense, to attack the colonists' settlements (Ostler, 2020). In both hard truths emanating from the Declaration of Independence, Whites had no appetite for ending Black enslavement and the genocide and dispossession perpetrated against the Indigenous people.

More recently, DiAngelo (2018) summarized the White colonists' deceptive and racist 1776 *Declaration of Independence*, the colonists' atrocities, and minority groups' responses vis-à-vis identity politics throughout American history as:

> The United States was founded on the principle that all people are created equal. Yet the nation began with the attempted genocide of Indigenous people and the theft of their land. American wealth was built on the labor of kidnapped and enslaved Africans and their descendants. Women were denied the right to vote until 1920, and black women were denied access to that right until 1964…We have yet to achieve our founding principle, but any gains we have made thus far have come through identity politics.

The White colonists unleashed an aggressive strategy of genocide, not attempted genocide, against American Indians. Barring the allusion to attempted genocide, DiAngelo's statement tells the story of the power and efficacy of identity politics, as a potent source and inspiration for racial minority groups to end racial oppression and attain freedom from modern slavery. In recent years, criticisms against identity politics from those who incorrectly posited that it represented the end of America (Churchwell, 2019), as indicated by a Federalist society tweet on October 2018, or the end of liberal democracy (Fukuyama, 2018), or that it started on the left, should peruse this definition of identity politics as: when people embrace political views grounded in their ethnicity/race, sexuality, or religion and not on comprehensive policy frameworks (Fukuyama, 2018). Thus, critics of identity politics should know that almost all significant events in American history owed their origins to identity politics (Churchwell, 2019).

To the amazement of critics of identity politics in the year 2020, the "Black Lives Matter" movement, an expression of identity politics, delivered potency and unification, not polarization, a strategic ingredient in the pursuit of equality and justice and ending White-imposed racism. Identity politics, energized through the added momentum of the national and international multiracial "Black Lives Matter" movement, is relevant and efficacious to challenge the unfulfilled ideals of liberty and justice for Americans of color linked to and a product of the deep-rooted problem of systemic racism and racial oppression in the country (Bobo, 2017). The systematic character of racial oppression demeans and dilutes the enormous Black historical content in the history of America, showing that Blacks inputted a huge portion of American history, from the duration of slavery of 246 years from 1619 to 1865, which is 60% of America's history; then reconstruction arose out of slavery for a brief period between 1865 and 1877, followed by 92 years of near slavery referred to as Jim Crow segregation. Slavery and the Jim Crow era constituted about 82% of American history. Yet, American history, for all intents and purposes, has been presented mainly as White history, in order to dilute the narrative on perpetual racial oppression and White-imposed racism against Blacks.

Systemic Racism

Racial oppression against Blacks and American Indians was embedded in the foundation of the first English Colony at Jamestown in 1607. This persisting racial oppression remains dominant in the early years of the twenty-first century because of systemic racism, which operates through the White racial frame. However, prior to exploring the "White racial frame" and "systemic racism," it is critical to review these concepts of "frame," "framing," and "frame analysis." Goffman saw frames as "schemata of interpretation" (Goffman, 1974, p. 21), whereby people may utilize frames as filters to acquire a sense of the world in which they live and the social events of the time. These frames also are situated at the structural level representing common beliefs of a society (Lowe, 2020). While people's behaviors are shaped by the collective frames (Benford & Snow, 2000), they will still make sense of the world around them through their own frame, but these frames will also comply with the dominant frame (Lowe, 2020). In the context of the USA, the dominant frame is the White racial frame.

But even with these explanations of the terms "frame" and "framing," the literature presents them as interchangeable with "ideology," when they are not (Benford & Snow, 2000; Oliver & Johnston, 2000). Following Oliver and Johnston (2000), framing has to do with process and ideology relates to content. This distinction between ideology and framing means that ideology delivers the content and background knowledge that people use to interpret a situation and framing enables people to utilize this ideology. Framing is rooted in ideology and can facilitate changes through resistance (Lowe, 2020). Nonetheless, in the first place, any effort aimed at societal transformation must first use a frame analysis to identify dominant frames, detecting how people frame their experiences through people's discourses in particular situations. Then, we can work backwards from the frame to understand and determine the ideological roots from which the frame evolved (Lowe, 2020). With this sense of frames, of framing, and of the link between framing and ideology, it is now timely to review the White racial frame and its connection to systemic racism. The White racial frame was embedded in the foundation of colonial America at the Jamestown settlement in 1607. Hence, America has been endowed with a racial structural foundation that is still part of its framework today. It is an America with systemic racial oppression, a history of hundreds of years of Native American genocide, hundreds of years of extreme oppression of African Americans, and decades of oppression against other communities of color.

Most recently, the awareness of systemic racism has gained momentum through the Black Lives Matter movement, police killings of Blacks (BBC, 2021)—Eric Garner on July 17, 2014; Michael Brown on August 9, 2014; Tamir Rice on November 22, 2014; Walter Scott on April 4, 2015; Alton Sterling on July 5, 2016; Philando Castile on July 6, 2016; Stephon Clark on March 18, 2018; Breonna Taylor on March 13, 2020; George Floyd on May 25, 2020; and Daunte Wright on April 11, 2021. And amid the ongoing COVID-19 pandemic, Blacks and other communities of color are experiencing demographic overrepresentation in cases, hospitalizations, and deaths.

The theorizing of the White racial frame and systemic racism, drawing from the Black counter-frame tradition (Ture et al., 1967) as well as the social sciences (Bonilla-Silva, 1997), arose from European imperialism and colonialism aimed at communities of color (Elias & Feagin, 2020a). In fact, systemic racism theory is rooted in the critical-race literature created during the 1960s Black civil rights movement and first enunciated for the health-care system by Ture et al. (1967). In their work, Ture and Hamilton posited that decisions and policies are grounded in racism, in order to subordinate a racial group. Earlier scholars and activists of color such as David Walker, Frederick Douglass, W.E.B. Du Bois, Anna Julia Cooper, Ida B. Wells-Barnett, and Oliver Cox laid the foundation for a developed structural and systemic racism paradigm (Feagin, 2020).

A roundtable discussion on the White racial frame presented Feagin's fundamental position on systemic racism theory (Bracey et al., 2017); thus: Feagin sees traditional race theories as overstating attitudes and individual characteristics, short of recognizing that racism is central to all American institutions; the traditional theories of race emphasize interpersonal and temporal actions, such as prejudice and discrimination, as the causal drivers of racial oppression; and he presents White racism as structural and recursive, since it is implanted in all social institutions.

Feagin (2001, pp. 5–6) defines systemic racism as:

> ...systemic racism includes the complex array of [discriminatory practices directed at people of color], the unjustly gained political-economic power of whites, continuing economic and other resource inequalities along racial lines, and white racist ideologies and attitudes created to maintain and rationalize white privilege and power. Systemic here means that the core racist realities are manifested in each of society's major parts...Each major part of U.S. society – the economy, politics, education, religion, the family – reflects the fundamental reality of systemic racism.

The key arguments of systemic racism are that it is mushrooming and that Whites are critical in the creation of racist societies, culminating in the formation of a color line separating the worlds of Whites and the people of color as a disadvantaged group (Elias & Feagin, 2020b). The strategic concepts in systemic racism theory (Feagin, 2020) are:

1. Dominant racial hierarchy.
2. The White racial frame: used to justify racial oppression, White privilege, and dominance over people of color, and seeing and interpreting the world through a White Eurocentric lens.
3. Individual and collective discrimination.
4. Social reproduction of inequalities predicated on racism.
5. Racist institutions fundamental to White domination of people of color.

These concepts of systemic racism theory offer a sense of the racial realities in the USA; thus:

> Much of the social terrain of this society is significantly racialized. Most major institutional and geographical space, acceptable societal norms, acceptable societal roles, privileged lan-

guage forms, preferred sociopolitical thinking, and favored understandings of history are white-generated, white-shaped, white-imposed, and/or white authenticated. All people, whether they are defined socially as white or not white, live largely within a substantially white-determined environment (Feagin, 2006, p. 47).

Clearly, COVID-19 is no great equalizer, as it is definitively increasing racial health disparities. Furthermore, it is common knowledge that Blacks and Whites are residentially segregated, with Blacks more likely to be residing in densely populated urban environments, more conducive to contracting COVID-19. Blacks and Whites are also occupationally segregated. The US Bureau of Labor Statistics (BLS, 2020) indicated that Blacks and Hispanics were demographically underrepresented in top-tier White-collar occupations/professions and demographically overrepresented in the essential services' occupations. Table 3.1 shows the underrepresentation of Blacks and Hispanics in top-tier professions. Clearly, Blacks and Hispanics are underrepresented among chief executives, surgeons, other physicians, dentists, paramedics, physician assistants, etc.

On the other hand, Table 3.2 shows the overrepresentation of Blacks and Hispanics in essential services' occupations that are conducive to contracting COVID-19. Blacks are demographically overrepresented in frontline occupations, such as nursing assistants, health technologists and technicians, bus drivers, etc., which are not amenable for workers to function virtually or remotely and to engage in social distancing measures.

The systemic racism perspective sees Whites and especially powerful Whites as primary agents in the creation and sustainability of White racist societies. Feagin (2020) noted that from its inception, America was built on racial oppression via systemic racism, facilitated by the White racial frame. In the early twentieth century, Du Bois (1920) noted that "Whiteness" had become a new religion in society, molded by the color line and racial hierarchies created by the dominant Whites.

Table 3.1 Distribution of Whites and minorities in White-collar occupations/professions

Occupations	Total employed	Women	2020 Percent of total employed White (%)	Black (%)	Asian (%)	Hispanic (%)
Total, 16 years and over	147,795	46.8	78.0	12.1	6.4	17.6
Chief Executives	1669	29.3	88.0	4.3	5.4	7.4
Surgeons	54	26.3	82.4	4.2	13.4	15.6
Other physicians	929	40.6	67.0	8.5	22.0	8.8
Dentists	173	28.7	78.8	1.4	16.6	5.5
Physician Assistants	141	65.5	79.9	6.3	12.3	7.9
Pharmacists	327	61.6	67.9	8.3	20.0	3.4
Registered Nurses	3257	87.4	75.3	13.4	8.7	7.9
Paramedics	78	28.1	93.2	3.9	2.8	8.5

Source for data: Adapted from BLS (2020)

Table 3.2 Distribution of Whites and minorities in essential services' occupations

| Occupations | Total employed | 2020 | | | | |
| | | Percent of total employed | | | | |
		Women (%)	White (%)	Black (%)	Asian (%)	Hispanic (%)
Total, 16 years and over	147,795	46.8	78.0	12.1	6.4	17.6
Nursing assistants	1364	89.3	57.0	35.2	4.7	13.7
Miscellaneous health technologists and technicians	185	61.7	57.8	24.8	15.3	13.5
Licensed practical and licensed vocational nurses	596	90.0	68.0	25.6	2.9	15.3
Bus drivers, transit and intercity	187	40.7	56.1	37.0	3.6	17.7
Couriers and messengers	578	22.6	69.9	21.1	4.4	23.1
Postal service clerks	91	62.1	49.5	38.4	9.6	10.2
Postal service mail carriers	312	36.7	72.7	18.7	6.8	13.6
Food servers, non-restaurant	157	77.1	68.6	18.8	7.7	22.0
Phlebotomists	101	84.8	66.0	27.6	2.8	9.0

Source for data: Adapted from BLS (2020)

An important function of the White racial frame is to belligerently encourage narratives portraying White superiority. The dominant White-created racial frame is a predominant Eurocentric worldview intersecting the divisions of class, race, gender, and age, becoming the frame of reference for Americans on racial matters (Feagin, 2020). The White racial frame includes beliefs (racial stereotypes, prejudices, and ideologies), cognition (racial interpretations and narratives), feelings (racialized emotions), and proclivity to action (discrimination). Together, these elements within the White racial frame constitute a hegemonic in-group superiority and an outgroup inferiority dominating the entire society (Feagin, 2020), not only at the interpersonal and internal levels but also at the systemic level through the major political, economic, and social institutions.

Feagin (2013) feels that at the individual level, subordinate groups could challenge the dominant White racial frame through "deframing," where an individual person can intentionally dissect a frame, in order to inspect all its components. Deframing may facilitate some "reframing," to create a new frame, so as to present an issue in a different way. He argues that when reframing occurs on a large scale, for example, via protest movements, it becomes counter-framing with a new collective action frame to resist the dominant White racial frame, manifested through anti-racist counter-frames and home-culture frames. He further suggests that the anti-racist counter-frame is a tool that racially oppressed groups use to challenge the dominant White racial frame, and that the home-culture frame is embedded in the ethnic culture of the group to create a new identity that could become antithetical to the dominant White racial frame.

A conclusive statement of Feagin's systemic racism theory would suggest the following: the White racial frame as a process enables people to develop a sense of the world through the content it draws from systemic racism as a racist ideology; the White racial frame mirrors both structural factors and institutional practices, in which health inequalities and inequities are rooted in American society; while supporting systemic racism, the White racial frame sustains racist systems and institutions vis-à-vis racist interpretations of the world. Systemic racism operates through the White racial frame.

Bonilla-Silva (2015) argued that Whites set up a social collectivity and cultivate a racial interest to preserve the racial status quo. The White racial status quo is the White racial frame. Thus, to end systemic racism requires effecting an end to the White racial frame. Like Feagin, Bonilla-Silva came out of the tradition of critical race research. Bonilla-Silva (2015) argued for a comprehensible theory on the modus operandi and institutionalization of racism. He sees race as a by-product of a system of racial domination where racism is more than a prejudice, more than an attitude or belief at the individual level because racism is rooted in the structure of American society. He introduced a different perspective to understand racism, referred to as racialized social systems, defined as being in "societies in which economic, political, social, and ideological levels are partially structured by the placement of actors in racial categories or races" (Bonilla-Silva, 2001, p.37). This racialization creates a genuine structure that places people in racial categories within a changing racial hierarchy, generating superordinate (top position) and subordinate (bottom position) social relations between the races. People at the top formulate views and practices supportive of the racial status quo, and people at the bottom take on views to challenge those positions articulated at the top level. This opposition between the races creates racial contestations. Thus, the way to figure out racism is "uncovering the mechanisms and practices (behaviors, styles, cultural affectations, traditions, and organizational procedures) at the social, economic, ideological, and political levels responsible for the reproduction of racial domination" (Bonilla-Silva, 2015, p.75).

Bonilla-Silva (1997) noted that people within racialized social systems have different life chances. The more disparate the racial groups' life chances, the greater the racialization of the social systems, and the more similar the racial groups' life chances, the less racialized the social systems. Bonilla-Silva posited that, historically, racialized social systems could also coexist with other types of oppression, as racialization happens in formations also structured by class and gender. However, the quality of racialized social systems may determine, too, whether class interests supersede racial interests or vice versa. For Blacks in American history, racial interests seem to have superseded class interests.

Nevertheless, the systemic prominence of class as it relates to race rises when the political, economic, and social distance between the races dwindle. Following Bonilla-Silva, the higher the inequality in society, the greater the racialized social systems, and lesser impact of class. The lesser the inequality in society, the lesser the racialized social systems, and the greater the impact of class. Among G7 countries, the USA had the highest income inequality at 41.4 Gini coefficient in 2018 (Bank, 2021). In 2019, the median wealth of Black households in the USA was $24,100 in comparison with $189,100 for White households (Weller & Roberts,

2021); the characteristic Black household had 12.7% of the wealth of the characteristic White household, and Blacks owned $165,000 less in wealth; and the average Black household earned $142,330 in 2019 in comparison with $980,549 for the average White household. Based on this data, the USA is a highly unequal society, with an increased level of racialized social systems.

America's highly racialized social system, the superiority complex of Whites as Du Bois (1920) noted, has been bolstered by numerous years of living in a White supremacist world. It has generated a deep Whiteness, prompting Bonilla-Silva to signal, "We cannot change the world of race if we do not know how deeply the practice of Whiteness has affected those we wish to transform" (Bonilla-Silva, 2015, p. 81).

There is a general consensus on three realities: racial stratification dates back to slavery; there is institutionalized racial discrimination with an overt Jim Crow framework in the South and a covert Jim Crow framework in the North; that the racial animus against Black Americans has social origins (Forman, 1972). But what is at stake is to determine an appropriate methodology to calculate how these three strategic realities are linked, how they function, and how they could be changed (Carmichael et al., 2003), in order to formulate a conceptual model for eliminating racism. The White racial frame inclusive of White-imposed racism (Feagin, 2020) and racialized social systems (Bonilla-Silva, 2001) link racial stratification, racial discrimination, and racial animus amid COVID-19.

Why a Focus on COVID-19 Deaths?

This study was necessary against the backdrop of the highly contagious COVID-19, which continues to expose White-imposed racism and racial oppression along with persisting racial health inequalities and inequities on Blacks and other communities of color in American society, notwithstanding progresses in public health, medical technology, and health care (Hummer, 1996). More particularly, despite COVID-19 has the capacity to infect anyone and everyone, that is, to be an equalizer, instead, the pathogen's conspicuous and demographically disproportionate impact on Blacks and other communities of color is compelling, but not surprising. The current racial and ethnic disparities in COVID-19 cases, hospitalizations, and deaths are evidence of systemic inequity, which is the "other pandemic" (Gray et al., 2020).

Blacks and Hispanics carry a demographic overrepresentation in cases and deaths, thus:

In Chicago, Illinois, rates of COVID-19 cases as per 100,000 as of June 1, 2020 were highest among Latino (2101.9) and "other" racial groups (1439.7), Black (1341.8), White (574.7), and Asian (557.7) residents. Mortality rates were highest among Black (120.5 per 100,000), Latino (81.6 per 100,000), Asian (57.3 per 100,000), and White (46.6 per 100,000) residents (CDPH, 2020). As of May 7, 2020, New York City presented a higher age-adjusted COVID-19 mortality among

Latino (187 per 100,000), Black (184 per 100,000), and White (93 per 100,000) residents (NYC Health, 2020).

Blacks and other historically racially disadvantaged groups have experienced demographic disproportionality in the burden of COVID-19 deaths, thereby increasing racial mortality. As of December 10, 2020, on age-standardized COVID-19 death rates with unweighted population distributions in the USA, Blacks had 22.60% of deaths, when they comprised 12.70% of the population, Hispanics carried a death rate of 36.30%, when they comprised 19.40% of the population, and Whites had a death rate of 32.80%, when they constituted 58.70% of the population (CDC, 2020a).

This significant racial mortality gap differed significantly across US States, counties, and neighborhoods, where such spatial variation was likely to indicate how place or urban-rural differences influence racial health disparities (O'Brien et al., 2020), as well as COVID-19 deaths. The urban-rural classification may also impact the sorts of and mode, through which the policies that spawn racial inequities are utilized, affecting health (Bell & Owens-Young, 2020). Likewise, an emphasis on urban-rural counties was strategic, since one in five US counties is disproportionately Black and they account for almost six of ten COVID-19 deaths throughout the USA (Millett et al., 2020).

We expect this study to throw light on the following questions:

- Given the urban-rural classification has been studied in population health and has been correlated with different indicators of structural racism in other contexts, how robust is this urban-rural classification in an analysis of COVID-19 deaths among Whites, Blacks, and Hispanics?
- Is there a social nexus between duality of structure in structuration theory and the White racial frame and racialized social systems as the platform, enabling a focus on a Black-White duality, in the search for pathways toward dismantling systemic racism?

Possible explanations for the demographic overrepresentation are:

- Racial/ethnic minorities and poor people experience demographic overrepresentation in underlying comorbidities, such as diabetes, cardiovascular disease, asthma, HIV, morbid obesity, liver disease, and kidney disease (Hooper et al., 2020).
- Susceptibility of poor Blacks is more than the impact of comorbidity. Yancy (2020), in a persuasive narrative, showed the vulnerability of poor Blacks to contracting COVID-19, which goes beyond comorbidity and thereby underscored the challenges the poor encounter vis-à-vis the mitigation measures. He noted that many Blacks lived in poor neighborhoods, with high housing density, high crime rates, and meager access to healthy foods and that low socioeconomic status by itself was a major risk factor for total mortality.

Hence, understanding the Black health experience and the Black health crisis along with the other people of color amid COVID-19 requires a critical examination of race as the significant variable in any true depiction of the US health-care system. Racial health disparities have been linked to the failure of the US health-care system. COVID-19 has exposed the racial health disparities and inequities in American society, imperatively necessitating an examination of the dynamics between systemic racism and the COVID-19 impact on Blacks and other people of color, in order to explore any association with COVID-19 deaths. This study reviewed six types of the urban and rural environments and their impact on COVID-19 deaths among Whites, Blacks, and Hispanics. In fact, among Blacks and underserved minority groups, racism continues to be a fundamental cause of diseases and the foundation of racial health inequities.

Drawing from the Malone-Heckler report in the 1980s, Byrd and Clayton (1992) identified the US health system's characteristics, thus: institutional and ideological race and class-based segregation and discrimination; race and class-based inequities and inequalities inherent in every molecule of the 375-year-old health system; and increased huge race and class-based health outcomes and health disparities. The Institute of Medicine report on differential treatment, while quite influential (IOM, 2003), never used the term "institutional racism" in its report (Feagin & Bennefield, 2014). But if nothing else is that good with the presence of the pandemic, paradoxically, COVID-19 brings into sharp focus the demographic overrepresentation of Blacks and other underserved minority groups in clinical outcomes—cases, hospitalizations, and deaths—vividly presenting the framework for unequal health risks in this way:

> The COVID-19 pandemic continues to deepen health disparities in our country. Long-standing inequalities have increased the risk for severe COVID-19 illnesses and death for many people. This both causes and continues disparities between racial and ethnic minority groups and non-Hispanic white people. Unequal health risks are the result of different conditions where people live, work, learn, play, and age—what we call social determinants of health (CDC, 2021b).

The CDC, by conceding that the long-standing and growing inequalities increased the risk of death from COVID-19, has affirmed the presence of the race and class-based segregation of health care in American society, one for the people of color and the other for Whites. Overall, the COVID-19 data for the country (NCHS/CDC, 2021) as of March 24, 2021, indicated that Hispanics were demographically overrepresented in the percentage of deaths at 31.8, when their population was 19.40%, and Blacks also were demographically overrepresented in the percentage of deaths at 22.30, when their population was 12.70%. These statistics, however, do reflect the age-old systemic racial health inequalities, and inequities responsible for exposing a huge number of people from racial and ethnic minority groups at increased risk of contracting and subsequently dying from COVID-19. Data on race and ethnicity in excess of 90% of COVID-19 deaths showed that the Hispanic or Latino, non-Hispanic Black, and non-Hispanic American Indian or Alaska Native people were disproportionately represented in the percentage of deaths, and this racial disparity worsens, when the percentages are age-standardized (CDC, 2020b).

Purpose of Study

The purpose of this study originated from the premise that the COVID-19 pandemic, just as the H1N1 pandemic, has conspicuously exposed the deeply embedded systemic racism that is the foundational reality of American society. The health inequity prominently prevailing is not new, and "…much of the inequity that spans generations results from poverty, structural racism, discrimination, and disinvestment in many communities of color" (Gracia, 2020, p. 518). Further, urban-rural differences have been studied in population health and were related to different indicators of systemic racism, so further exploring the role of urban-rural classification was necessary. Hence, the first purpose of this study was to explore whether demographic overrepresentation of COVID-19 deaths among Whites, Blacks, and Hispanics varied by urban-rural classification and whether urban-rural classification was an independent risk factor for COVID-19 deaths among communities of color.

> "Over the past half-century, understanding of health and healthcare disparities in the United States — including underlying social, clinical, and system-level contributors — has increased. Yet disparities persist. Eliminating health disparities will require a movement away from disparities as the focus of research and toward a research agenda centered on achieving racial equity by dismantling structural racism" (Lavizzo-Mourey et al., 2021, p. 1681).
>
> And so, the second purpose was to review the social nexus between duality of structure in structuration theory and the White racial frame and racialized social systems as the platform and a focus on a Black-White duality, in the search of pathways toward dismantling systemic racism.

Studies on Racial Health Disparities Amid COVID-19

Selected Literature

Due to the *SpringerBrief* guidelines limiting the size of the manuscript, we present only a few selected findings to show that Blacks and other people of color in relation to their White counterparts are demographically overrepresented in COVID-19 cases, hospitalizations and deaths. We have used search strategy COVID-19 AND (morbidity OR mortality) AND (Blacks OR Hispanics OR Native Americans) for Embase and PsycINFO databases, PubMed for identifying systematic reviews on racial health disparities amid COVID-19 for the period January 1, 2020 through January 31, 2021. We identified 12 papers, of which five (5) studies were included and seven (7) excluded, as they were not relevant to the primary outcome of this study. To identify literature on Blacks with comorbidity amid COVID-19, we used this search term for PubMed: *comorbidities and COVID-19 among Black Americans* (96 results, 6 used). For additional papers, we also used Google Scholar for the period "since 2020" with these general search terms: *racial health disparities*; *comorbidity in COVID-19, ethnicity; blacks, COVID-19 infections and mortality*; *poverty responsible for contracting COVID-19*; *COVID-19 mortality and comorbidity by race/ethnicity*; and identified articles from references. To be clear, we were unable to include several papers in this selected literature.

COVID-19 places everyone at risk and anyone without immunity to this highly contagious pathogen is vulnerable. There is this erroneous assumption that all persons will equally be impacted by the virus (Mein, 2020). This group of medical comorbidities, such as diabetes, hypertension, cardiovascular disease, and obesity among Blacks has created the environment for viruses like COVID-19 to flourish and cause severe infections. Some risk mitigation measures, such as mobility restrictions, physical distancing, hygienic measures, socioeconomic restrictions, communication and international support mechanisms, cordons sanitaire, traffic restriction, home quarantine, centralized quarantine, and a mixture of voluntary and enforceable tools, have been critical as primary prevention measures to contain the contagion spread, along with testing some measures to see whether they would produce positive outcomes as they did for SARS (Nussbaumer-Streit et al., 2020; Wilder-Smith & Freedman, 2020; Wells et al., 2020; Bruinen de Bruin et al., 2020; Pan et al., 2020a). Even though these mitigation measures were introduced to flatten the curve, reduce the spread of the pathogen, and limit the pressure on healthcare facilities, these suggestions unintentionally preferentially harm the socially disadvantaged (Mein, 2020).

Yancy (2020), in a compelling narrative, showed the susceptibility of poor Blacks to contracting COVID-19 that goes beyond comorbidity and thereby underscored the challenges the poor encounter vis-à-vis the mitigation measures. However, when infected, the socially disadvantaged were at a higher risk for increased disease severity (Mein, 2020), as comorbidities have an association with severe influenza illness (Blumenshine et al., 2008). COVID-19 patients with severe symptoms, who also have other comorbidities like hypertension, diabetes, chronic obstructive pulmonary disease (COPD), heart diseases, malignancies, and HIV, were associated with significant morbidity and mortality (Ejaz et al., 2020). Epidemiological studies found that these comorbidity conditions were prevalent among racial/ethnic minorities and other socially disadvantaged populations, probably resulting in poorer COVID-19 outcomes (Hutchins et al., 2009).

The COVID-19 pandemic in the USA has thrown an enormous glare of spotlight on health disparities among people of color in relation to incidence, morbidity, hospitalizations, and mortality. Generally, disparities could lead to a disproportionately greater prevalence of disease or reduced standard of care given to the index group. Several studies, among others (Raine et al., 2020; Gu et al., 2020; Alcendor, 2020; Abedi et al., 2020; Kopel et al., 2020; Kim & Bostwick, 2020; Gross et al., 2020; Tartof et al., 2020; Moore et al., 2020; Rogers et al., 2020; Vahidy et al., 2020b; Reed, 2021; Li et al., 2020; Kullar et al., 2020; Holtgrave et al., 2020), have presented a demographic overrepresentation of Blacks and other people of color in COVID-19 cases, morbidity, hospitalizations, and deaths. Hence, for this limited literature review, we selected a few papers on racial health disparities in clinical outcomes amid COVID-19.

A commentary on racial health disparities (Kirksey et al., 2021) suggested that Blacks, who comprised some 12.8% of the US population suffered the most and had the highest death rates. Several factors were advanced to explain the plight of Blacks and other communities of color in this pandemic: (1) inadequate availability of testing; (2) a remarkable increase in low wage worker unemployment/health insurance loss, particularly, in the service sector of the economy; (3) high rates of preexisting chronic disease conditions like, diabetes, hypertension, coronary artery disease, kidney disease, cancer, and stroke, among others; (4) limited access to early health care; and (5) single provider and structural health care system bias. "Indeed, COVID-19 represents a pandemic superimposed on a historic epidemic of racial health inequity and healthcare disparities" (Kirksey et al., 2021, p. 39).

On the basis of 13 cross-sectional and cohort studies, this systematic review (Mackey et al., 2020) found that Blacks experienced disproportionately higher infection rates and excess mortality, but not higher case fatality rates; Hispanics suffered disproportionately higher infection rates and excess mortality, but not higher case-fatality rates; and Blacks experienced 1.5–3.5 times higher risk of contracting the SARS-CoV-2 infection. Six ecological and two serological studies also supported the finding that Blacks experienced a higher rate of SARS-CoV-2 infection. The review also reported that Hispanics had a 1.3–7.7 times higher risk of becoming infected with COVID-19 compared to Whites. According to Mackey et al. (2020), racial health disparities could be the result of exposure-related factors such as population density and inadequate access to health care, and not susceptibility (comorbidity), which may be discrepancies within the ethnic strata contributing to poverty, but they are insufficient to explain racial health disparities. Population density in poor neighborhoods, limited access to health care, high crime rates, and insufficient access to healthy foods may very well be characteristics of low socioeconomic status (SES), a key risk factor for total mortality (Yancy, 2020) and other types of susceptibility to COVID-19. SES may induce or be the cause of health inequalities, but racial health inequalities persist not because of SES, but because racism is an essential cause of racial differences in SES (Phelan & Link, 2015).

The Bronx Montefiore Health System's COVID-19 study revealed that Blacks had a higher mortality with COVID-19, incompletely explicated by age, comorbidities, and metrics relating to sociodemographic disparities (Golestaneh et al., 2020), and these researchers (2020 p. 7) concluded that:

> The COVID pandemic has unmasked a disparity in health outcomes. We cannot be sure of its biologic significance, but it seems to be real and present in the Black community beyond the usual explanations of clinical comorbidities and easily available socioeconomic factors. The possibility that unrecognized severity of comorbidity or social vulnerability because of pre-pandemic unequal access to care, or differential failure to remediate those recognized comorbidities/social vulnerabilities, cannot be excluded.

The exposure factors were further supported by a major study in Houston (Vahidy et al., 2020a) that showed that population density had some relationship to infection rates for Blacks, and also, population density and income accounted for infection rates for Hispanics. In addition, a study on multihospital health-care system in Southern California (Ebinger et al., 2020), in defining the demographic and clinical characteristics of comorbidities/preexisting conditions, concluded that they were largely products of social and economic disadvantage, which resulted in greater severity of COVID-19 infection among people of color. However, preexisting conditions and vulnerability to contracting infections, while relevant for any discussion of COVID-19, have been used in public health research to obscure huge absolute racial health disparities.

In addition, a retrospective cohort study (Ogedegbe et al., 2020) conducted within the New York University Langone Health system found that Black and Hispanic populations were not innately more susceptible to developing poor COVID-19 outcomes than other groups and that if they became hospitalized, they progressed as well as or better than their White counterparts. These researchers inferred that the higher mortality observed in Black populations could fundamentally be explained through higher out-of-hospital deaths, as a result of the lower neighborhood SES in the Black communities. This finding championed the claim that existing structural determinants, such as inequality in housing, access to care, differential employment opportunities, and poverty that persisted in Black and Hispanic communities require active interventions, to reverse the outrages historically disadvantaged people of color have been enduring for centuries. Another study (Poulson et al., 2021) called for a better knowledge of the racial health disparities of COVID-19, in order to adequately speak to the root causes. Those racial roots have lineage to the founding of America. Racial health disparities have been gawking Americans in their faces since 1619, yet the Poulson study predicated the need for better understanding of racial health disparities with an appreciation of its origins. That mindset has limited interest in solving America's race problems, a mindset that sustains the White racial frame and color-blind racism.

However, susceptibility to COVID-19 has become an attractive topic for research during this pandemic, due to its disproportionate impact on people of color. It is almost as if using "susceptibility" is the easy way out to explain the plight of Blacks and other communities of color in this pandemic. An observational cohort study during the first phase of the pandemic (March 5, 2020–June 7, 2020) (Pflugeisen & Mou, 2020) evaluated the association between ethnicity and outcomes of coronavirus positivity and hospitalization and found that people of color, especially Latinx (18.6%), were more probable to test positive for COVID-19. For Latinx patients, 18. 6% of those tested were positive compared to a positivity of 4.0% for the tested White patients. Many people of color in this study (Pflugeisen & Mou, 2020) had limited health insurance coverage and limited capacity to engage in social distancing, working remotely, etc., and so experienced increased susceptibility to viral exposure. These findings are consistent with those in a Washington, DC, study (Martinez et al., 2020).

A Massachusetts study (Hu et al., 2020) assessed racial segregation and disparities in testing site access, utilizing economic, demographic, and transportation variables at the city/town level. The study found that higher Black segregations with high housing densities of more than one occupant per room and a rising poverty rate were probably correlated with high COVID-19 incidence rate. This finding was consistent with the Washington State study (Pflugeisen & Mou, 2020). In the same vein, a cross-sectional study (Figueroa et al., 2020) reviewed specific demographic, economic, and occupational factors to determine their inputs to disparities in

COVID-19 incidence rates across Massachusetts. People of color were found to be susceptible to the COVID-19 disease, and this disadvantaged population seemed to be a prominent predictor in this cross-sectional study of 351 Massachusetts cities and towns from January 1, 2020 to May 6, 2020. Then there was the study on 31,549 adults tested for COVID-19 between March 1, 2020 and July 10, 2020 in Milwaukee and southeast Wisconsin (Egede et al., 2020), which also revealed overrepresentation of historically disadvantaged groups with positivity status for COVID-19. The study alluded to structural racism, residential segregation, and social risk in the USA and their inputs to poor health outcomes as explanations for their findings.

Demographic overrepresentation of ethnic minority groups with COVID-19 positivity status was found, too, in an observational study (Wang et al., 2020) within the Mount Sinai Health System in New York City (Bronx, Brooklyn, Manhattan, Queens, and Staten Island). The study found that Hispanics (29%) and African Americans (25%) had disproportionately high positive case rates relative to their numbers in the New York City population. The study advanced the view that differences in positivity may be the outcome of true differences in infection rates, quite consistent with greater case density in places as Brooklyn and Queens, with huge populations of Blacks and Hispanics (USCB, 2020), and a low neighborhood SES, quite consistent with Yancy's position of "Where and how black individuals live matters. If race per se enters this discussion, it is because in so many communities, race determines home" (Yancy, 2020, p. 1891). A US and UK study (Sze et al., 2020), the first meta-analysis containing 50 papers, to probe the association between ethnicity and clinical outcomes in COVID-19, found that Blacks and Asians experienced a higher risk of becoming infected with SARS-CoV-2 than White patients, whereas the Asian patients faced a higher risk of intensive therapy unit (ITU) admission and possible death due to their contraction of severe COVID-19 pneumonia. The study explained that the disproportionate impact of COVID-19 on Black and Asian patients may be attributable to the higher rates of infection in their communities, similar to the Wang et al. (2020) study.

A cohort study (Yehia et al., 2020) comprised 11,210 adult patients (age $\geq$ 18 years) hospitalized with confirmed SARS-CoV-2 from February 19, 2020 through May 31, 2020 in 92 hospitals in 12 states: Alabama (6 hospitals), Maryland (1 hospital), Florida (5 hospitals), Illinois (8 hospitals), Indiana (14 hospitals), Kansas (4 hospitals), Michigan (13 hospitals), New York (2 hospitals), Oklahoma (6 hospitals), Tennessee (4 hospitals), Texas (11 hospitals), and Wisconsin (18 hospitals). The study found similar all-cause in-hospital mortality for hospitalized White 23.1% (724 of 3218) and Black patients 19.2% (540 of 2812). After controlling for age, sex, insurance, comorbidities, neighborhood deprivation, and site of care, there was no statistically significant difference in risk of mortality between Black and White patients. Notwithstanding that numerous findings indicated that Blacks were demographically overrepresented in COVID-19 infections and deaths in the USA (Yancy, 2020), what do we make of this finding of no difference in risk of mortality for both Black and White patients? Could it be that Blacks were hospitalized in larger numbers than Whites? The largest Black populations are in 10 States (New York, California, Texas, Florida, Georgia, Illinois, North Carolina, Maryland,

Michigan, and Louisiana), of which the Yehia et al. study only covered five (New York, California, Texas, Florida and Georgia) of those 10 States, which had more than 2 million Blacks each.

Medical comorbidities seemed to be a driver of the disproportionality among the racially disadvantaged in COVID-19 mortality (Pan et al., 2020b). But COVID-19 morbidity and mortality were worsened vis-à-vis racial health disparities, occupational hazard, and poverty in New York City (Arasteh, 2020), where these conditions together induced greater rates at which the disadvantaged people of color became exposed to COVID-19, and the prevalence of comorbidities made them susceptible, where critical care was essential to fight COVID-19 compounded by their comorbidities. Also, when infected, the poor people of color seemed to be at a higher risk for increased disease severity (Mein, 2020), as comorbidities had a link with severe influenza illness (Blumenshine et al., 2008).

A multinational meta-analysis study, with 54 studies from the USA and 15 from the UK (Raharja et al., 2020), found reliable evidence of the racially disadvantaged groups disproportionately sharing COVID-19 morbidity and mortality. The study concluded that racial health disparities may be related to higher rates of medical comorbidities. Nevertheless, even if comorbidities may be linked to racial overrepresentation in COVID-19 mortality, then what environments are breeding grounds for the development of medical comorbidities? A focus on the environment would necessitate consideration of exposure and access to health-care variables within the overall intersectional framework of social class, race, and gender.

Methods

Study Design

This research used the theory-informing inductive data analysis study design (Varpio et al., 2020) to explore the nationwide, 14-State, and 5-State COVID-19 deaths among Whites, Blacks, and Hispanics. This inductive research entailed moving from specific data relating to a particular experience to a general conceptualization of that experience, that is, a bottom-up approach, and this study did not commence with a hypothesis. The subjectivist inductive research design, as outlined by Varpio et al., contains two assumptions: one, the social construction of the reality is uneven, as it exists because people share a provisional conceptual framework on the multiple interpretations and multiple perceptions of a reality, and two, to really develop a sense of the reality necessitates walking around the preexisting de-identified data. A tentative conceptual framework emerged during the study as new ideas, insights, and knowledge was advanced. Accordingly, the White racial frame (Feagin, 2020) was advanced in this chapter, recognizing that it would be adjusted as data began to transform the COVID-19 impact. Hence, the rollout of the data analysis preceded formulation of theories to explain data interpretations.

Data Collection

The motivation for this study arose out of the characteristic mounting racial health disparities in the current COVID-19 pandemic, with astounding similarities to previous epidemics and pandemics. Indeed, the current public health emergency bringing with it total exposure of racial inequities and inequalities did not surprise Americans. Again, as during previous diseases, communities of color have remained the most susceptible and vulnerable to the pathogen, and availability of race/ethnic data remained typically lethargic and incomplete during this pandemic. So it was not surprising that a Congressional letter of March 27, 2020 was sent to the Former United States Secretary of Health and Human Services Honorable Alex M. Azar II, signed by Senator Elizabeth Warren, Representative Ayanna Pressley, Representative Robin L. Kelly, former Senator Kamala D. Harris (now US Vice President), and Senator Corey A. Booker (Warren et al., 2020, pp. 1, 3) to ensure that appropriate race and ethnic data was available.

This study analyzed provisional data on COVID-19 deaths in 760 Counties in 50 States and the District of Columbia (excluding territories outside mainland USA), among Whites, Blacks, and Hispanics, mainly utilizing this CDC dataset:

- National provisional deaths by county, and race/ethnicity (CDC, 2021a). This dataset did not provide complete data for all the counties in each State. For instance, here is an illustration of a few States with data availability only for some of their counties: New York State has 62 counties, but data was provided only for 31 counties; California has 58 counties, but data was available only for 34 counties; Texas has 254 counties, but data was only provided for 52 counties; while Florida has 67 counties, data was provided only for 36 counties; Georgia has 159 counties, but data was available only for 42 counties; and while Illinois has 102 counties, data was available only for 26 counties.

We utilized several other CDC datasets, including the NCHS on health disparities relating to provisional COVID-19 death count, COVID-19 mortality overview, and the CDC data tracker, along with the Kaiser Family Foundation (KFF).

County data on race and Hispanic origin were extracted from 760 counties in 50 States and DC; this dataset contains only counties with more than 100 COVID-19 deaths (CDC, 2021a). The urban-rural classification in this study complied with the 2013 National Center for Health Statistics Urban-Rural Classification Scheme for Counties (https://www.cdc.gov/nchs/data_access/urban_rural.htm, last accessed on 20 June 2021). This study used the dataset on COVID-19 deaths cumulative from week-ending January 4, 2020, to April 17, 2021.

Analyses focused on the 50 States and DC in relation to the following variables:

Dependent Variable

COVID-19 Deaths Among Whites, Blacks, and Hispanics.

CDC (2018) defines provisional data on deaths as preliminary data, based on new and updated records from States. Provisional data may be issued monthly or quarterly and are subject to change as information is constantly being collected and analyzed. CDC presents provisional data as estimates that may be at variance with the final count. The CDC has noted that the provisional counts for COVID-19 deaths are sourced from the National Vital Statistics System (NVSS). The national provisional counts consisted of COVID-19 deaths within the 50 States and DC. The CDC signaled that several weeks may elapse prior to the submission of death records to the NCHS, to be processed, coded, and tabulated. Death counts for previous weeks are frequently revised, resulting in an increase or decrease, as new and updated death certificate data is obtained from the States by NCHS. The CDC further noted that COVID-19 death counts as indicated in this dataset may be at variance with other data sources, since there is presently a lagging of data by an average of 1–2 weeks.

Independent Variables

State/County: Urban/Rural, based on the six urbanization levels of the 2013 NCHS Urban-Rural Classification (metropolitan [large central metro, large fringe metro, medium metro, small metro] and nonmetropolitan [micropolitan, noncore]). Figure 3.1 shows the classification scheme.

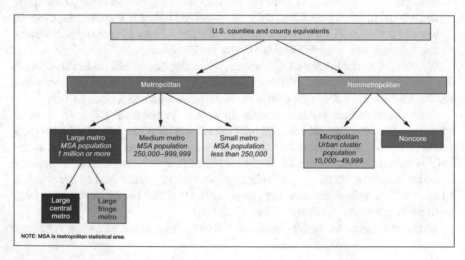

Fig. 3.1 Structure of the 2013 NCHS urban–rural classification scheme for counties. (Source: CDC 2014)

Metropolitan Counties

Large central metro counties in metropolitan statistical areas (MSA) of 1 million population that:

1. comprise the whole population of the largest principal city of the MSA; or
2. are entirely enclosed within the largest principal city of the MSA; or
3. have at least 250,000 residents of any principal city in the MSA.

   Large fringe metro counties in MSA of 1 million or more population, but are not eligible to be as large as central.

   Medium metro counties in MSA of 250,000–999,999 population. *Small metro counties* are counties in MSAs with less than 250,000 population.

Nonmetropolitan Counties

These are micropolitan counties in micropolitan statistical areas, and noncore counties not within micropolitan statistical areas.

It is common knowledge that State-level statistics do not provide a full picture of racial health disparities, since several US States are also acutely segregated. What this means is that different counties in the same State may deliver hugely different breakdowns by race and ethnicity and, also, some counties have a different racial/ethnic image from their own States.

Research Questions

- After comparing the means of COVID-19 deaths among Whites, Blacks, and Hispanics across the six types of independent urban-rural counties (large central metro, large fringe metro, medium metro, small metro, micropolitan, and noncore), was there statistical evidence that the related population means were significantly different in the COVID-19 deaths among Whites, Blacks, and Hispanics across the urban-rural counties?
- Did COVID-19 deaths among Whites, Blacks, and Hispanics differ by urban-rural classification nationwide?
- Did COVID-19 deaths among Whites, Blacks, and Hispanics differ by urban-rural classification in the 14 States with the largest Black and Hispanic populations (Arizona, California, Colorado, Florida, Georgia, Illinois, Louisiana, Maryland, New Jersey, New Mexico, New York, North Carolina, Texas, Virginia)?

- Did COVID-19 deaths among Whites, Blacks, and Hispanics differ by urban-rural classification in the top five (5) States of residence for the US Black population (Texas, Florida, Georgia, New York, and California)?
- Was the urban-rural classification an independent risk factor for COVID-19 deaths among Whites, Blacks, and Hispanics?
- Which counties had the greatest effect on COVID-19 deaths among Whites, Blacks, and Hispanics?
- Is there a social nexus between duality of structure in structuration theory and the White racial frame as the platform, enabling a focus on the Black-White paradigm, in the search for theoretical pathways toward dismantling systemic racism?

Statistical Measures

1. Descriptive statistics on urban and rural States/counties by COVID-19 deaths among Whites, Blacks, and Hispanics.
2. Testing for significance between States/counties (independent variable) and COVID-19 deaths among Whites, Blacks, and Hispanics (dependent variables).

SPSS Statistics 25 facilitated the processing and analysis of the de-identified data (CDC, 2021a). The study applied these statistical protocols: descriptive statistics, Kruskal-Wallis Test, Dunn's Post Hoc Test, and using the Bonferroni correction. The tests used a significance level of $p<0.05$.

Ethics Approval

For this study, we used publicly available data that did not contain any personal information, so no ethical review was obligatory. Patients or the public were not engaged in the design, or conduct, or reporting, or dissemination plans of our study. This study did not involve human subjects as defined in 45 CFR 46. The analysis utilized preexisting de-identified aggregated publicly available data. Thus, it is classified as a study of non-human subjects research.

References

Abedi, V., Olulana, O., Avula, V., Chaudhary, D., Khan, A., Shahjouei, S., Li, J., & Zand, R. (2020). Racial, economic and health inequality and COVID-19 infection in the United States. *medRxiv*.
Alcendor, D. J. (2020). Racial disparities-associated COVID-19 mortality among minority populations in the US. *Journal of Clinical Medicine, 9*.

Arasteh, K. (2020). Prevalence of comorbidities and risks associated with COVID-19 among black and Hispanic populations in new York City: An examination of the 2018 new York City Community health survey. *Journal of Racial and Ethnic Health Disparities.*

Bank, W. (2021). *Gini index (World Bank estimate) [online].* World Bank. Available: https://data.worldbank.org/indicator/SI.POV.GINI. Accessed 1 July 2021

BBC. (2021). *George Floyd: Timeline of black deaths and protests* [online]. BC. Available: https://www.bbc.com/news/world-us-canada-52905408. Accessed 22 Apr 2021.

Beck, A. F., Edwards, E. M., Horbar, J. D., Howell, E. A., Mccormick, M. C., & Pursley, D. M. (2020). The color of health: How racism, segregation, and inequality affect the health and well-being of preterm infants and their families. *Pediatric Research, 87,* 227–234.

Bell, C. N., & Owens-Young, J. L. (2020). Self-rated health and structural racism indicated by county-level racial inequalities in socioeconomic status: The role of urban-rural classification. *Journal of Urban Health, 97,* 52–61.

Benford, R. D., & Snow, D. A. (2000). Framing processes and social movements: An overview and assessment. *Annual Review of Sociology, 26,* 611–639.

BLS. (2020). *Employed persons by detailed occupation, sex, race, and Hispanic or Latino ethnicity* [online]. U.S. Bureau of Labor Statistics. Available: https://www.bls.gov/cps/cpsaat11.pdf. Accessed 22 Apr 2021.

Blumenshine, P., Reingold, A., Egerter, S., Mockenhaupt, R., Braveman, P., & Marks, J. (2008). Pandemic influenza planning in the United States from a health disparities perspective. *Emerging Infectious Diseases, 14,* 709.

Bobo, L. D. (2017). Racism in Trump's America: Reflections on culture, sociology, and the 2016 US presidential election. *The British Journal of Sociology, 68,* S85–S104.

Bonilla-Silva, E. (1997). Rethinking racism: Toward a structural interpretation. *American Sociological Review*, 465–480.

Bonilla-Silva, E. (2001). *White supremacy and racism in the post-civil rights era.* Lynne Rienner Publishers.

Bonilla-Silva, E. (2015). More than prejudice: Restatement, reflections, and new directions in critical race theory. *Sociology of Race and Ethnicity, 1,* 73–87.

Boyd, R. W., Lindo, E. G., Weeks, L. D., & Mclemore, M. R. (2020). On racism: A new standard for publishing on racial health inequities. *Health Affairs Blog, 10.*

Bracey, G., Chambers, C., Lavelle, K., & Mueller, J. C. (2017). *The white racial frame: A roundtable discussion. Systemic Racism.* Springer.

Bruinen De Bruin, Y., Lequarre, A. S., Mccourt, J., Clevestig, P., Pigazzani, F., Zare Jeddi, M., Colosio, C., & Goulart, M. (2020). Initial impacts of global risk mitigation measures taken during the combatting of the COVID-19 pandemic. *Safety Science, 104773.*

Byrd, W. M., & Clayton, L. A. (1992). An American health dilemma: A history of blacks in the health system. *Journal of the National Medical Association, 84,* 189.

Carmichael, S., Thelwell, M., Wideman, J. E., & Ture, K. (2003). *Ready for revolution: The life and struggles of Stokely Carmichael (Kwame Ture).* Simon and Schuster.

CDC. (2014). *2013 NCHS urban–rural classification scheme for counties* [online]. DHHS. Available: https://www.cdc.gov/nchs/data/series/sr_02/sr02_166.pdf. Accessed 1 May 2021.

CDC. (2018). *Understanding Death Data* [Online]. CDC. Available: https://www.cdc.gov/surveillance/projects/understanding-death-data.html. Accessed 2 May 2021].

CDC. (2020a). *COVID-19 racial and ethnic health disparities* [online]. CDC. Available: https://www.cdc.gov/coronavirus/2019-ncov/community/health-equity/racial-ethnic-disparities/disparities-deaths.html. Accessed 14 June 2021.

CDC. (2020b). *COVID-19 racial and ethnic health disparities* [online]. CDC. Available: https://www.cdc.gov/coronavirus/2019-ncov/community/health-equity/racial-ethnic-disparities/disparities-deaths.html. Accessed 18 Mar 2021.

CDC. (2021a). *Provisional COVID-19 death counts by county and race* [online]. CDC. Available: https://data.cdc.gov/NCHS/Provisional-COVID-19-Death-Counts-by-County-and-Ra/k8wy-p9cg/data. Accessed 14 Apr 2021.

CDC. (2021b). *The unequal toll of the COVID-19 pandemic* [online]. CDC. Available: https://www.cdc.gov/coronavirus/2019-ncov/covid-data/covidview/. Accessed 14 Mar 2021.

CDPH. (2020). *Report date: June 01, 2020* [online]. Chicago Department of Public Health. Available: https://www.chicago.gov/city/en/sites/covid-19/home/latest-data.html. Accessed 20 Apr 2021.

Chowkwanyun, M. (2011). The strange disappearance of history from racial health disparities research. *DuBois Review, 8*, 253–270.

Churchwell, S. (2019). *America's original identity politics*. The New York Review.

Diangelo, R. (2018). *White fragility: Why it's so hard for white people to talk about racism*. Beacon Press.

Du Bois, W. (1920). *2003, The souls of white folk* (pp. 17–18). Darkwater: Voices Behind the Veil, Prometheus.

Du Bois, W. E. B. (2008). *The souls of black folk*. Oxford University Press.

Ebinger, J. E., Achamallah, N., Ji, H., Claggett, B. L., Sun, N., Botting, P., Nguyen, T. T., Luong, E., Kim, E. H., Park, E., Liu, Y., Rosenberry, R., Matusov, Y., Zhao, S., Pedraza, I., Zaman, T., Thompson, M., Raedschelders, K., Berg, A. H., … Cheng, S. (2020). Pre-existing traits associated with Covid-19 illness severity. *PLoS One, 15*, e0236240.

Egede, L. E., Walker, R. J., Garacci, E., Raymond, S. R., & J. R. (2020). Racial/ethnic differences in COVID-19 screening, hospitalization, and mortality in Southeast Wisconsin: Study examines racial/ethnic differences in COVID-19 screening, symptom presentation, hospitalization, and mortality among 31,549 adults tested for COVID-19 in Wisconsin. *Health Affairs, 39*, 1926–1934.

Ejaz, H., Alsrhani, A., Zafar, A., Javed, H., Junaid, K., Abdalla, A. E., Abosalif, K. O., Ahmed, Z., & Younas, S. (2020). COVID-19 and comorbidities: Deleterious impact on infected patients. *Journal of Infection and Public Health*.

Elias, S., & Feagin, J. R. (2020a). *Systemic racism and the white racial frame* (pp. 12–29). Routledge International Handbook of Contemporary Racisms.

Elias, S., & Feagin, J. R. (2020b). *Systemic racism and the white racial frame*. Routledge International Handbook of Contemporary Racisms.

Feagin, J. R. (2001). *Racist America: Roots, current realities, and future reparations*. Routledge.

Feagin, J. R. (2006). *Systemic racism: A theory of oppression*.

Feagin, J. R. (2013). *The white racial frame: Centuries of racial framing and counter-framing*. New York, Routledge.

Feagin, J. R. (2020). *The white racial frame: Centuries of racial framing and counter-framing*. Routledge.

Feagin, J., & Bennefield, Z. (2014). Systemic racism and US health care. *Social Science & Medicine, 103*, 7–14.

Figueroa, J. F., Wadhera, R. K., Lee, D., Yeh, R. W., & Sommers, B. D. (2020). Community-level factors associated with racial and ethnic disparities in COVID-19 rates in Massachusetts: Study examines community-level factors associated with racial and ethnic disparities in COVID-19 rates in Massachusetts. *Health Affairs, 39*, 1984–1992.

Forman, J. (1972). *The making of black revolutionaries*. University of Washington Press.

Fukuyama, F. (2018). Can liberal democracies survive identity politics? *The Economist, 30*.

Garcia, M. A., Homan, P. A., García, C., & Brown, T. H. (2020). The color of COVID-19: Structural racism and the pandemic's disproportionate impact on older racial and ethnic minorities. *The Journals of Gerontology: Series B*.

Goffman, E. (1974). *Frame analysis: An essay on the organization of experience*. Harvard University Press.

Golestaneh, L., Neugarten, J., Fisher, M., Billett, H. H., Gil, M. R., Johns, T., Yunes, M., Mokrzycki, M. H., Coco, M., & Norris, K. C. (2020). The association of race and COVID-19 mortality. *EClinicalMedicine, 25*, 100455.

Gracia, J. N. (2020). COVID-19's disproportionate impact on communities of color spotlights the Nation's systemic inequities. *Journal of Public Health Management and Practice, 26*, 518–521.

Gray, D. M., Anyane-Yeboa, A., Balzora, S., Issaka, R. B., & May, F. P. (2020). COVID-19 and the other pandemic: Populations made vulnerable by systemic inequity. *Nature Reviews Gastroenterology & Hepatology, 17*, 520–522.

Gross, C. P., Essien, U. R., Pasha, S., Gross, J. R., Wang, S. Y., & Nunez-Smith, M. (2020). Racial and ethnic disparities in population-level Covid-19 mortality. *Journal of General Internal Medicine, 35*, 3097–3099.

Gu, T., Mack, J. A., Salvatore, M., Prabhu Sankar, S., Valley, T. S., Singh, K., Nallamothu, B. K., Kheterpal, S., Lisabeth, L., Fritsche, L. G., & Mukherjee, B. (2020). Characteristics associated with racial/ethnic disparities in COVID-19 outcomes in an academic health care system. *JAMA Network Open, 3*, e2025197.

Guasco, M. (2017). *The Fallacy of 1619: Rethinking the History of Africans in Early America* [Online]. Available: https://www.aaihs.org/the-fallacy-of-1619-rethinking-the-history-of-africans-in-early-america/. Accessed 25 Oct 2020.

Hammonds, E. M., & Reverby, S. M. (2019). *Toward a historically informed analysis of racial health disparities since 1619*. American Public Health Association.

Hardeman, R. R. (2020). Examining racism in health services research: A disciplinary self-critique. *Health Services Research, 55*, 777.

Holtgrave, D. R., Barranco, M. A., Tesoriero, J. M., Blog, D. S., & Rosenberg, E. S. (2020). Assessing racial and ethnic disparities using a COVID-19 outcomes continuum for New York State. *Annals of Epidemiology, 48*, 9–14.

Hooper, M. W., Nápoles, A. M., & Pérez-Stable, E. J. (2020). COVID-19 and racial/ethnic disparities. *JAMA, 323*, 2466–2467.

Hu, T., Yue, H., Wang, C., She, B., Ye, X., Liu, R., Zhu, X., Guan, W. W., & Bao, S. (2020). Racial segregation, testing site access, and COVID-19 incidence rate in Massachusetts, USA. *International Journal of Environmental Research and Public Health, 17*, 9528.

Hummer, R. A. (1996). Black-white differences in health and mortality: A review and conceptual model. *The Sociological Quarterly, 37*, 105–125.

Hutchins, S. S., Fiscella, K., Levine, R. S., Ompad, D. C., & Mcdonald, M. (2009). Protection of racial/ethnic minority populations during an influenza pandemic. *American Journal of Public Health, 99*, S261–S270.

IOM. (2003). *Unequal treatment: Confronting racial and ethnic disparities in health care*. The National Academies Press.

Jefferson, T. (1776). Declaration of independence: A transcription. *National Archives, 4*.

Kim, S. J., & Bostwick, W. (2020). Social vulnerability and racial inequality in COVID-19 deaths in Chicago. *Health Education & Behavior, 47*, 509–513.

Kirksey, L., Tucker, D. L., Taylor, E., Jr., White Solaru, K. T., & Modlin, C. S., Jr. (2021). Pandemic superimposed on epidemic: Covid-19 disparities in black Americans. *Journal of the National Medical Association, 113*, 39–42.

Kopel, J., Perisetti, A., Roghani, A., Aziz, M., Gajendran, M., & Goyal, H. (2020). Racial and gender-based differences in COVID-19. *Frontiers in Public Health, 8*, 418.

Kullar, R., Marcelin, J. R., Swartz, T. H., Piggott, D. A., Macias Gil, R., Mathew, T. A., & Tan, T. (2020). Racial disparity of coronavirus disease 2019 in African American communities. *The Journal of Infectious Diseases, 222*, 890–893.

Lavizzo-Mourey, R. J., Besser, R. E., & Williams, D. R. (2021). Understanding and mitigating health inequities—Past, current, and future directions. *New England Journal of Medicine, 384*, 1681–1684.

Li, D., Gaynor, S. M., Quick, C., Chen, J. T., Stephenson, B. J. K., Coull, B. A., & Lin, X. (2020). Unraveling US national COVID-19 racial/ethnic disparities using county level data among 328 million Americans. *medRxiv*.

Lowe, R. J. (2020). *The 'native Speaker' Frame: Establishing a theoretical framework. Uncovering Ideology in English Language Teaching*. Springer.

Mackey, K., Ayers, C. K., Kondo, K. K., Saha, S., Advani, S. M., Young, S., Spencer, H., Rusek, M., Anderson, J., Veazie, S., Smith, M., & Kansagara, D. (2020). Racial and ethnic disparities in COVID-19-related infections, hospitalizations, and deaths: A systematic review. *Annals of Internal Medicine*.

Martinez, D. A., Hinson, J. S., Klein, E. Y., Irvin, N. A., Saheed, M., Page, K. R., & Levin, S. R. (2020). SARS-CoV-2 positivity rate for Latinos in the Baltimore–Washington, DC region. *JAMA, 324*, 392–395.

Mccord, C., & Freeman, H. P. (1990). Excess mortality in Harlem. *New England Journal of Medicine, 322*, 173–177.

Mckay, D. L., Vinyeta, K., & Norgaard, K. M. (2020). Theorizing race and settler colonialism within US sociology. *Sociology Compass, 14*, e12821.

Mein, S. A. (2020). COVID-19 and health disparities: The reality of "the great equalizer". *Journal of General Internal Medicine, 35*, 2439–2440.

Millett, G. A., Jones, A. T., Benkeser, D., Baral, S., Mercer, L., Beyrer, C., Honermann, B., Lankiewicz, E., Mena, L., Crowley, J. S., Sherwood, J., & Sullivan, P. S. (2020). Assessing differential impacts of COVID-19 on black communities. *Annals of Epidemiology, 47*, 37–44.

Moore, J. T., Ricaldi, J. N., Rose, C. E., Fuld, J., Parise, M., Kang, G. J., Driscoll, A. K., Norris, T., Wilson, N., Rainisch, G., Valverde, E., Beresovsky, V., Agnew Brune, C., Oussayef, N. L., Rose, D. A., Adams, L. E., Awel, S., Villanueva, J., Meaney-Delman, D., & Honein, M. A. (2020). Disparities in Incidence of COVID-19 Among Underrepresented Racial/Ethnic Groups in Counties Identified as Hotspots During June 5–18, 2020–22 States, February–June 2020. *MMWR. Morbidity and Mortality Weekly Report, 69*, 1122–1126.

NCHS/CDC. (2021). *COVID-19 racial and ethnic health disparities* [online]. NCHS, CDC. Available: https://www.cdc.gov/coronavirus/2019-ncov/community/health-equity/racial-ethnic-disparities/disparities-deaths.html. Accessed 28 Mar 2021.

Nussbaumer-Streit, B., Mayr, V., Dobrescu, A. I., Chapman, A., Persad, E., Klerings, I., Wagner, G., Siebert, U., Christof, C., Zachariah, C., et al. (2020). Quarantine alone or in combination with other public health measures to control COVID-19: A rapid review. *Cochrane Database of Systematic Reviews*.

NYC Health. (2020). *COVID-19: Data [Online]*. NYC Health. Available: https://www1.nyc.gov/site/doh/covid/covid-19-data.page. Accessed 20 Apr 2021

O'brien, R., Neman, T., Seltzer, N., Evans, L., & Venkataramani, A. (2020). Structural racism, economic opportunity and racial health disparities: Evidence from US counties. *SSM-Population Health, 11*, 100564.

Ogedegbe, G. (2020). Responsibility of medical journals in addressing racism in health care. *JAMA Network Open, 3*, –e2016531.

Ogedegbe, G., Ravenell, J., Adhikari, S., Butler, M., Cook, T., Francois, F., Iturrate, E., Jean-Louis, G., Jones, S. A., Onakomaiya, D., Petrilli, C. M., Pulgarin, C., Regan, S., Reynolds, H., Seixas, A., Volpicelli, F. M., & Horwitz, L. I. (2020). Assessment of racial/ethnic disparities in hospitalization and mortality in patients with COVID-19 in new York City. *JAMA Network Open, 3*, e2026881.

Oliver, P., & Johnston, H. (2000). What a good idea! Ideologies and frames in social movement research. *Mobilization: An International Quarterly, 5*, 37–54.

Ostler, J. (2020). *The Shameful Final Grievance of the Declaration of Independence* [Online]. Available: https://www.theatlantic.com/ideas/archive/2020/02/americas-twofold-original-sin/606163/. Accessed 22 Oct 2020.

Pan, A., Liu, L., Wang, C., Guo, H., Hao, X., Wang, Q., Huang, J., He, N., Yu, H., Lin, X., Wei, S., & Wu, T. (2020a). Association of Public Health Interventions with the epidemiology of the COVID-19 outbreak in Wuhan, China. *JAMA*, e206130.

Pan, D., Sze, S., Minhas, J. S., Bangash, M. N., Pareek, N., Divall, P., Williams, C. M., Oggioni, M. R., Squire, I. B., Nellums, L. B., Hanif, W., Khunti, K., & Pareek, M. (2020b). The impact of ethnicity on clinical outcomes in COVID-19: A systematic review. *EClinicalMedicine, 23*, 100404.

Pflugeisen, B. M., & Mou, J. (2020). Empiric evidence of ethnic disparities in coronavirus positivity in Washington state. *Ethnicity & Health*, 1–13.

Phelan, J. C., & Link, B. G. (2015). Is racism a fundamental cause of inequalities in health? *Annual Review of Sociology, 41*, 311–330.

Pirtle, W. N. L. (2020). Racial capitalism: A fundamental cause of novel coronavirus (COVID-19) pandemic inequities in the United States. *Health Education & Behavior.*

Poulson, M., Geary, A., Annesi, C., Allee, L., Kenzik, K., Sanchez, S., Tseng, J., & Dechert, T. (2021). National Disparities in COVID-19 outcomes between black and white Americans. *Journal of the National Medical Association, 113*, 125–132.

Raharja, A., Tamara, A., & Kok, L. T. (2020). Association between ethnicity and severe COVID-19 disease: A systematic review and meta-analysis. *Journal of Racial and Ethnic Health Disparities*, 1–10.

Raine, S., Liu, A., Mintz, J., Wahood, W., Huntley, K., & Haffizulla, F. (2020). Racial and ethnic disparities in COVID-19 outcomes: Social determination of health. *International Journal of Environmental Research and Public Health, 17.*

Reed, D. D. (2021). Racial disparities in healthcare: How COVID-19 ravaged one of the wealthiest African American counties in the United States. *Social Work in Public Health, 36*, 118–127.

Rogers, T. N., Rogers, C. R., Vansant-Webb, E., Gu, L. Y., Yan, B., & Qeadan, F. (2020). *Racial disparities in COVID-19 mortality among essential Workers in the United States.* World Med Health Policy.

Serchen, J., Doherty, R., Atiq, O., & Hilden, D. (2020). Racism and health in the United States: A policy statement from the American College of Physicians. *Annals of Internal Medicine, 173*, 556–557.

Sze, S., Pan, D., Nevill, C. R., Gray, L. J., Martin, C. A., Nazareth, J., Minhas, J. S., Divall, P., Khunti, K., Abrams, K. R., Nellums, L. B., & Pareek, M. (2020). Ethnicity and clinical outcomes in COVID-19: A systematic review and meta-analysis. *EClinicalMedicine, 29*, 100630.

Tartof, S. Y., Qian, L., Hong, V., Wei, R., Nadjafi, R. F., Fischer, H., Li, Z., Shaw, S. F., Caparosa, S. L., Nau, C. L., Saxena, T., Rieg, G. K., Ackerson, B. K., Sharp, A. L., Skarbinski, J., Naik, T. K., & Murali, S. B. (2020). Obesity and mortality among patients diagnosed with COVID-19: Results from an integrated health care organization. *Annals of Internal Medicine, 173*, 773–781.

Ture, K., Hamilton, C. V., & Hamilton, C. V. (1967). *Black power: The politics of liberation* (pp. 63–64).

USCB. (2020). *QuickFacts: United States* [Online]. Available: https://www.census.gov/quickfacts/fact/table/US/PST045219. Accessed 21 Apr 2020.

Vahidy, F. S., Nicolas, J. C., Meeks, J. R., Khan, O., Pan, A., Jones, S. L., Masud, F., Sostman, H. D., Phillips, R., & Andrieni, J. D. (2020a). Racial and ethnic disparities in SARS-CoV-2 pandemic: Analysis of a COVID-19 observational registry for a diverse US metropolitan population. *BMJ Open, 10*, e039849.

Vahidy, F. S., Nicolas, J. C., Meeks, J. R., Khan, O., Pan, A., Jones, S. L., Masud, F., Sostman, H. D., Phillips, R., Andrieni, J. D., Kash, B. A., & Nasir, K. (2020b). Racial and ethnic disparities in SARS-CoV-2 pandemic: Analysis of a COVID-19 observational registry for a diverse US metropolitan population. *BMJ Open, 10*, e039849.

Varpio, L., Paradis, E., Uijtdehaage, S., & Young, M. (2020). The distinctions between theory, theoretical framework, and conceptual framework. *Academic Medicine, 95*, 989–994.

Wang, Z., Zheutlin, A., Kao, Y.-H., Ayers, K., Gross, S., Kovatch, P., Nirenberg, S., Charney, A., Nadkarni, G., & DE Freitas, J. K. (2020). Hospitalised COVID-19 patients of the Mount Sinai health system: A retrospective observational study using the electronic medical records. *BMJ Open, 10*, e040441.

Warren, E., Pressley, A., Kelly, R. L., Harris, K. D., & Booker, C. A. (2020). *Lawmakers urge HHS to address racial disparities in access to testing and treatment during the coronavirus pandemic*. Congress of the United States.

Weller, C. E. & Roberts, L. (2021). *Eliminating the black-white wealth gap is a generational challenge* [Online]. Available: https://www.americanprogress.org/issues/economy/reports/2021/03/19/497377/eliminating-black-white-wealth-gap-generational-challenge/. Accessed 1 July 2021.

Wells, C. R., Sah, P., Moghadas, S. M., Pandey, A., Shoukat, A., Wang, Y., Wang, Z., Meyers, L. A., Singer, B. H., & Galvani, A. P. (2020). Impact of international travel and border control measures on the global spread of the novel 2019 coronavirus outbreak. *Proceedings of the National Academy of Sciences of the United States of America, 117*, 7504–7509.

Wilcox, W. F. (1904). *The Negro Population* [Online]. Washington, DC: Bureau of the Census. Available: https://www2.census.gov/prod2/decennial/documents/03322287no8ch1.pdf [Accessed November 1, 2021].

Wilder-Smith, A., & Freedman, D. O. (2020). Isolation, quarantine, social distancing and community containment: Pivotal role for old-style public health measures in the novel coronavirus (2019-nCoV) outbreak. *Journal of Travel Medicine, 27*, taaa020.

Williams, D. R., Lawrence, J. A., & Davis, B. A. (2019). Racism and health: Evidence and needed research. *Annual Review of Public Health, 40*, 105–125.

Yancy, C. W. (2020). COVID-19 and African Americans. *JAMA, 323*(19), 1891–1892. https://doi.org/10.1001/jama.2020.6548

Yearby, R. (2020). Structural racism and health disparities: Reconfiguring the social determinants of health framework to include the root cause. *The Journal of Law, Medicine & Ethics, 48*, 518–526.

Yehia, B. R., Winegar, A., Fogel, R., Fakih, M., Ottenbacher, A., Jesser, C., Bufalino, A., Huang, R. H., & Cacchione, J. (2020). Association of Race with Mortality among patients hospitalized with Coronavirus Disease 2019 (COVID-19) at 92 US hospitals. *JAMA Network Open, 3*, e2018039.

Chapter 4
COVID-19 Deaths

The highly transmissible COVID-19 pandemic is not the great equalizer. This, certainly, doesn't sound like a message with any semblance of rationality because the pandemic is capable of infecting anyone and everyone, yet the virus has been disproportionately targeting the poor and vulnerable people of color in the USA. For instance, for the period of February 12, 2020–May 18, 2020, among 52,166 deaths from 47 jurisdictions, 55.4% were male, 79.6% were aged ≥65, 21.0% were Black, and 40.3% were White (Wortham et al., 2020). Yancy (2020), in his work on racial health disparities, focusing on differences in disease risk and fatality rates, cited these findings: In Michigan, Blacks accounted for 33% of COVID-19 cases and 40% of deaths, but constituted 14% of the population (Thebault et al., 2020). In Chicago, in excess of 50% of COVID-19 cases and about 70% of COVID-19 deaths were attributed to Blacks, notwithstanding that Blacks constituted only 30% of the population (Reyes et al., 2020). In Louisiana, Blacks accounted for 70.5% of deaths and constituted 32.2% of the State's population (AP, 2020). In New York City (NYC), Blacks and Hispanics had 28% and 34% of deaths, respectively, and constituted 22% and 29% of the NYC population, respectively (NYSDoH, 2020).

For this study, the CDC (2021) provided the dataset on the national provisional deaths by county, urban-rural, and race/ethnicity in the USA from January 1, 2020, through April, 17, 2021. Data collection on COVID-19 deaths complied with the 2013 National Center for Health Statistics Urban-Rural Classification Scheme for Counties (https://www.cdc.gov/nchs/data_access/urban_rural.htm, last accessed June 16, 2021).

As of June 2, 2021, COVID-19 deaths (age standardized with unweighted distribution of population) (NCHS/CDC, 2021) showed the following: Whites, 32.70% deaths, representing a population of 58.70%; Blacks, 22.50% deaths, representing a population of 12.70%; and Hispanics, 36.60% deaths, constituting some 19.40% of the population. Table 4.1 shows that COVID-19 deaths, unadjusted for age with unweighted distribution of population, for 760 counties within 50 States and DC (the CDC dataset did not carry data on COVID-19 deaths for all counties in the US,

P. Misir, *COVID-19 and Health System Segregation in the US*, Springer Briefs in Public Health, https://doi.org/10.1007/978-3-030-88766-7_4

Table 4.1 Descriptive statistics on COVID-19 deaths nationwide (January 1, 2020, to April 17, 2021)

Statistics

		State	County Name	Urban Rural Code	COVID-19 Deaths	White	Black	AI/AN	Hispanic
N	Valid	760	760	760	760	758	500	80	409
	Missing	0	0	0	0	2	260	680	351
Mean				3.19	650.20	377.62768	150.96747	59.80820	242.47406
Std. Error of Mean				.046	46.294	17.852608	13.056790	13.619602	38.789288
Median				3.00	275.00	203.50650	59.22700	21.98100	43.00800
Mode				2	105	66.045	13.038[a]	12.028	9.900[a]
Std. Deviation				1.264	1276.247	491.514433	291.958706	121.817426	784.464793
Variance				1.598	1628805.616	241586.437	85239.886	14839.485	615385.012
Range				5	21904	5177.016	3013.812	914.726	12026.879
Minimum				1	101	10.098	9.828	9.415	9.856
Maximum				6	22005	5187.114	3023.640	924.141	12036.735
Sum			2421		494153	286241.785	75483.735	4784.656	99171.889

a. Multiple modes exist. The smallest value is shown

Source: CDC (2021)

as data was compiled only for a county that had 100 or more COVID-19 deaths) from January 1, 2020 through April 17, 2021 were as follows: deaths among Whites were 286,242 (58%), constituting circa 60.10% of the population, with 144.9 deaths per 100,000; Blacks with 75,484 deaths (15%) constituting some 12.50% of the population, with 184.1 deaths per 100,000; and Hispanics with 99,172 deaths (20%) constituting some 18.50% of the population, with 162.5 deaths per 100,000. The range of total COVID-19 deaths in the 760 counties was 21,904 (4%), with 22,005 (4 percent) as the maximum and 101 as the minimum.

Looking at the aggregate data, the median number of deaths was less than or equal to 275 in half the total number of counties and the number of deaths was greater than 275 in half the total number of counties. The median number of deaths among Whites was less than or equal to 204 in half the total number of counties and the number of deaths was greater than 204 in half the total number of counties. The median number of deaths among Hispanics was less than or equal to 43 in half the total number of counties and the number of deaths was greater than 43 in half the total number of counties, and the median number of deaths among Blacks was less than or equal to 59 in half the total number of counties and the number of deaths was greater than 59 in half the total number of counties.

Table 4.2 shows that data on all-cause deaths was available for 760 counties within 50 States and DC. Here are some findings on race/ethnic groups on all-cause deaths in 760 counties: all-cause deaths among Whites were 2,510,539 (70%); Hispanics, 380,210 (11%); American Indians/Alaska Natives (AI/AN), 21,705 (0.006); and Asians, 114,998 (3%), and they were all demographically underrepresented. However, Blacks at 508,383 (14%) carried a disproportionate share of all-cause deaths. The way to measure the impact of a pandemic is through excess deaths, which is defined "…as the number of persons who have died from all causes, in excess of the expected number of deaths for a given place and time" (Rossen

Table 4.2 Descriptive statistics on all-cause deaths nationwide (January 1, 2020, to April 17, 2021)

Descriptive statistics

	N	Minimum	Maximum	Sum	Mean	
	Statistic	Statistic	Statistic	Statistic	Statistic	Std. error
Urban-rural code	760	1	6	2421	3.19	0.046
All-cause deaths	760	489	110,631	3,571,930	4699.91	261.828
White	760	11.99	42150.41	2510539.44	3303.3414	144.30512
Black	760	0.00	21138.74	508383.80	668.9260	56.91142
AI/AN	760	0.00	2097.83	21704.51	28.5586	4.42287
Asian	760	0.00	14824.55	114998.11	151.3133	26.05967
Hispanic	760	0.00	38499.59	380209.91	500.2762	73.74889
Valid N (listwise)	760					

Source: CDC (2021)

et al., 2020, p. 1522). Generally, an estimated 299,028 cxccss deaths appeared from late January through October 3, 2020, with 198,081 (66%) excess deaths credited to COVID-19 (Rossen et al., 2020). Almost 300,000 additional people died between January and October 2020 than would be expected in the similar time period in the years 2015 through 2019, and some two-thirds of these excess deaths were attributable to COVID-19. Relating to these excess deaths, Whites had the smallest growth at 11.9%; the biggest percentage growth (53.6%) was among Hispanics, their excess deaths largely attributable to COVID-19 deaths, as they were demographically underrepresented among all-cause deaths. There were excess deaths of 28.9% to 36.6% among Blacks and Asians, respectively. However, Blacks were the only group with a demographically disproportionate share of COVID-19 deaths in the three metrics: COVID-19 deaths, all-cause deaths, and excess deaths.

Urban-Rural Counties as Independent Risk Factors for COVID-19 Deaths

One of the research questions in this study was to compare the means of COVID-19 deaths among White, Black, and Hispanic across the six types of independent urban-rural counties (large central metro, large fringe metro, medium metro, small metro, micropolitan, and noncore), in order to conclude whether there was statistical evidence that the related population means were significantly different in the COVID-19 deaths among White, Black, and Hispanic across the urban-rural counties. Since the data, invariably, was not normally distributed, ANOVA (analysis of variance) could not be applied. Hence, the Kruskal-Wallis Test, the non-parametric equivalent to the one-way ANOVA, was used. The following assumptions for using Kruskal-Wallis Test have been met: (1) samples are random, (2) samples are typical of the populations, (3) samples are independent of each other, (4) dependent variable is a continuous random variable, and (5) distributions of the populations are similar in shape. The Kruskal-Wallis Test compared the median COVID-19 deaths among the White, Black, and Hispanic groups across the six types of urban-rural counties nationwide (50 States and DC).

Nationwide Urban-Rural Counties and COVID-19 Deaths

Hypotheses for the Kruskal-Wallis Test on the nationwide data:
The null hypothesis (H_0):

1. There were no differences in the median COVID-19 deaths among White, Black, and Hispanic across the six types of urban-rural counties nationwide.

The alternative hypothesis (H_1):

2. There were differences in the median COVID-19 deaths among White, Black, and Hispanic across the six types of urban-rural counties nationwide.

The Kruskal-Wallis Test was administered to evaluate differences ($p < 0.05$) in median COVID-19 deaths nationwide overall among Whites, Blacks, and Hispanics across six types of urban-rural counties (large central metro (county 1), large fringe metro (county 2), medium metro (county 3), small metro (county 4), micropolitan (county 5), and noncore (county 6)). The results of the Kruskal-Wallis chi-squared test were significant, H (5) = 300.871, p = 0.000, as the p-value was less than α (0.05). Hence, we rejected the null hypothesis and concluded that there were differences in median COVID-19 deaths of Whites, Blacks, and Hispanics among the six urban and rural counties nationwide.

The pairwise post hoc Dunn test ($p < 0.05$, adjusted using the Bonferroni correction) (Fig. 4.1) determined that the following pairs of counties were statistically significant ($p < 0.05$) on COVID-19 deaths overall among Whites, Blacks, and Hispanics nationwide: 6–4, noncore-small metro; 6–2, noncore-large fringe metro; 6–3, noncore-medium metro; 6–1, noncore-large central metro; 5–4, micropolitan-small metro; 5–2, micropolitan-large fringe metro; 5–3, micropolitan-medium metro; 5–1, micropolitan-large central metro; 4–2, small metro-large fringe metro; 4–3, small metro-medium metro; 3–1, medium metro-large central metro; 2–1, large fringe-metro-large central metro; and 4–1, small metro-large central metro. The nationwide data showed that the large central metro county seemed to have the greatest impact on COVID-19 deaths overall among Whites, Blacks, and Hispanics nationwide.

Disaggregating the nationwide data by White, Black, and Hispanic groups showed that the Kruskal-Wallis chi-squared test results of each group were significant, thus: Whites, H (5) = 234.642, p = 0.000; Blacks, H (5) = 110.024, p = 0.000; and Hispanics, H (4) = 86.052, p = 0.000, as the p-values were < α (0.05), indicating differences in median COVID-19 deaths for each group across the six types of urban-rural counties. The pairwise post hoc Dunn test ($p < 0.05$, adjusted using the

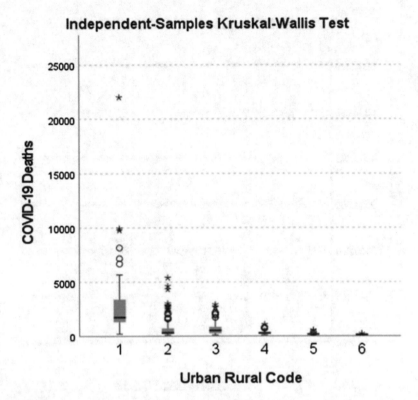

Fig. 4.1 COVID-19 deaths overall among Whites, Blacks, and Hispanics across urban-rural counties nationwide. (Source: CDC, 2021)

Bonferroni correction) identified the following pairs of counties as statistically significant on COVID-19 deaths among each group of Whites, Blacks, and Hispanics: Whites (Fig. 4.2): 6–2; 6–3; 6–1; 5–4; 5–2; 5–3; 5–1; 4–2; 4–3; 4–1; 2–1; and 3–1. Blacks (Fig. 4.3): 6–1; 4–2; 4–1; 5–1; 2–1; and 3–1. Hispanics (Fig. 4.4): 5–3; 5–2; 5–1; 4–3; 4–2; 4–1; 3–1; and 2–1. The disaggregated nationwide data analysis showed that the large fringe metro county had the greatest impact on COVID-19 deaths among Whites, the large central metro with a strong effect on COVID-19 deaths among Blacks and Hispanics.

Fourteen States: Urban-Rural Counties and COVID-19 Deaths

We then reviewed some selected descriptive statistics from January 1, 2020, through April 17, 2021, on COVID-19 deaths in 14 States with the largest Black and Hispanic populations (Arizona, California, Colorado, Florida, Georgia, Illinois,

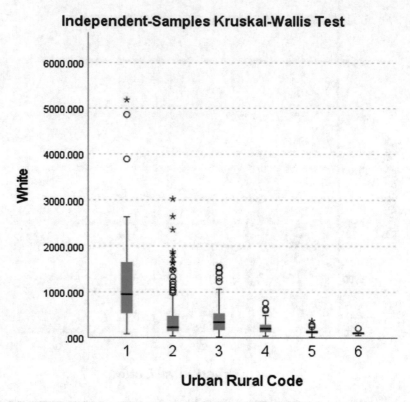

Fig. 4.2 COVID-19 deaths—Whites, nationwide. (Source: CDC, 2021)

Louisiana, Maryland, New Jersey, New Mexico, New York, North Carolina, Texas, Virginia).

Table 4.3 shows that about half of COVID-19 deaths nationwide happened in the large fringe metro (25%) and the medium metro (24%). Of the 14 States, Blacks were demographically overrepresented in COVID-19 deaths in the following nine (9) States: Florida, Georgia, Illinois, Louisiana, Maryland, New Jersey, North Carolina, Virginia, and New York. And Hispanics carried a disproportionate share in COVID-19 deaths in these four (4) States: California, Colorado, Texas, and New York.

We then used the Kruskal-Wallis Test to compare the median COVID-19 deaths among Whites, Blacks, and Hispanics across the six types of urban-rural counties in the 14 States.

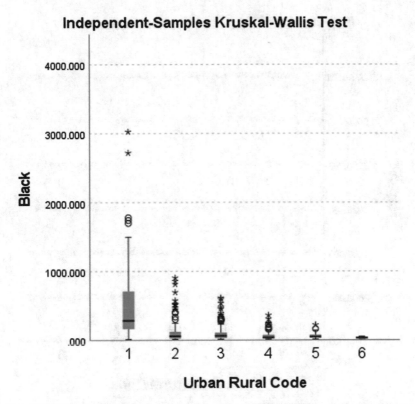

Fig. 4.3 COVID-19 deaths—Blacks, nationwide. (Source: CDC, 2021)

The null hypothesis (H$_0$):

1. There were no differences in the median COVID-19 deaths among Whites, Blacks, and Hispanics across the six types of urban-rural counties in the 14 States.

The alternative hypothesis (H$_1$):

2. There were differences in the median COVID-19 deaths among Whites, Blacks, and Hispanics across the six types of urban-rural counties in the 14 States.

Pertaining to the 14 States, the results of the Kruskal-Wallis chi-squared test were significant, H (5) = 134.555, p = 0.000, as the p-value was less than α (0.05). Hence, we rejected the null hypothesis and concluded that there were differences in median COVID-19 deaths overall among Whites, Blacks, and Hispanics across the six urban-rural counties in the 14 States.

The pairwise post hoc Dunn test (p < 0.05, adjusted using the Bonferroni correction) (Fig. 4.5) determined the following pairs of counties as statistically significant on COVID-19 deaths among Whites, Blacks, and Hispanics in the 14 States: 5–4;

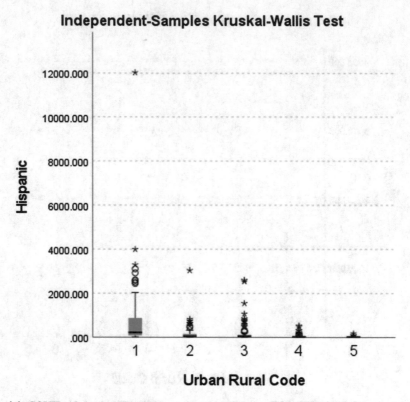

Fig. 4.4 COVID-19 deaths—Hispanics, nationwide. (Source: CDC, 2021)

5–3; 5–2; 5–1; 4–3; 4–1; 2–1; and 3–1. The 14 States' data showed that the large central metro county seemed to have the greatest impact on COVID-19 deaths of Whites, Blacks, and Hispanics combined.

Disaggregating data from 14 States on COVID-19 deaths by Whites, Blacks, and Hispanics, the Kruskal-Wallis chi-squared test results were significant, as their p-values were $< \alpha$ (0.05), thus: Whites, H (4) =103.114, p = 0.000; Blacks, H (4) =68.739, p = <0.001; and Hispanics, H (4) = 48.865, p = <0.001. Hence, there were differences in median COVID-19 deaths of each group among the six types of urban-rural counties in the 14 States.

The pairwise post hoc Dunn test (p < 0.05, adjusted using the Bonferroni correction) recognized that the following pairs of counties were statistically significant on COVID-19 deaths among each group in the 14 States: Whites (Fig. 4.6): 5–4; 5–3; 5–2; 5–1; 4–3; 4–1; 2–1; and 3–1. Blacks (Fig. 4.7): 5–1; 2–1; 3–1; 4–1; and 4–2. Hispanics (Fig. 4.8): 5–2; 5–3; 5–1; 4–1; 2–1; and 3–1. The 14 States' data analysis showed that the large fringe metro county had the greatest impact on COVID-19 deaths among Whites, and the large central metro with a strong effect on COVID-19 deaths among Blacks and Hispanics.

Table 4.3 COVID-19 deaths by race, 14 States, and urban-rural counties (January 1, 2020–April 17, 2021)

States	% COVID-19 deaths (% of population)[1]			Maximum % of deaths in urban and rural environments
	White	Black	Hispanic	
Nationwide	58 (60)	15 (13)	20 (19)	~half from both the large fringe metro (25%), and medium metro (24%)
California	31 (37)	6 (7)	48 (39)	38% from the medium metro
Colorado	64 (68)	5 (5)	26 (22)	~three-quarters from the large fringe metro (36%) and the medium metro (36%)
Florida	55 (53)	17 (17)	26 (26)	42% from the medium metro
Georgia	56 (52)	35 (33)	5 (10)	41% from the large fringe metro
Illinois	58 (61)	19 (15)	18 (18)	31% from the large fringe metro
Louisiana	55 (58)	40(33)	3 (5)	43% from the small metro
Maryland	51 (50)	36 (31)	9 (11)	63% from the large fringe metro
New Jersey	57 (55)	16 (15)	20 (21)	62% from the large fringe metro
New Mexico	25 (37)	0.009 (3)	38 (49)	43% from the small metro
North Carolina	63 (63)	27 (22)	6 (10)	38% from the medium metro
Arizona	51 (54)	3 (5)	31 (32)	46% from the small metro
Texas	40 (41)	10 (13)	47 (40)	31% from the large fringe metro
Virginia	60 (61)	26 (20)	8 (10)	45% from the large fringe metro
New York	47 (55)	21 (18)	22 (19)	Almost half are from the large fringe metro (26%) and the large central metro (23%)

(Source: CDC, 2021)
Note: [1](USCB, 2019)

Five States: Urban-Rural Counties and COVID-19 Deaths

Analysis of each of the top five (5) States of residence for the US Black population (Texas, Florida, Georgia, New York, and California) was conducted to establish whether there were no differences in the individual distribution of COVID-19 deaths of Whites, Blacks, and Hispanics among the urban-rural counties (H_0) or whether there were differences (H_1).

Table 4.4 shows that the Kruskal-Wallis chi-squared test results were significant in the 5 States for each group of Whites, Blacks, and Hispanics (except Blacks in California and Hispanics in Georgia), as their p-values were $< \alpha$ (0.05). Hence, we rejected the null hypothesis and concluded that there were differences in median COVID-19 deaths for each group among the six types of urban-rural counties in New York, Texas, and Florida; we also rejected the null hypothesis and concluded that there were differences in the median COVID-19 deaths for Whites and Blacks in Georgia, and only for Whites and Hispanics in California among the urban-rural counties.

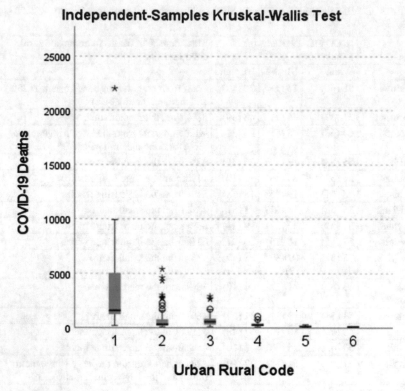

Fig. 4.5 COVID-19 deaths—overall among Whites, Blacks, and Hispanics in urban-rural counties in 14 States. (Source: CDC, 2021)

The pairwise post hoc Dunn test ($p < 0.05$, adjusted using the Bonferroni correction) recognized the following pairs of counties as statistically significant on COVID-19 deaths among Whites, Blacks, and Hispanics in each of the five States:

- New York—Whites (Fig. 4.9): 5–2; 5–1. Blacks (Fig. 4.10): 4–1; 3–1. Hispanics (Fig. 4.11): 3–1.
- Texas—Whites (Fig. 4.12): 5–4; 5–1; 2–1. Blacks (Fig. 4.13): 5–1; 4–1; 2–1. Hispanics (Fig. 4.14): 5–3; 5–1; 2–1; 4–1.
- Florida—Whites (Fig. 4.15): 4–1. Blacks (Fig. 4.16): 4–1. Hispanics (Fig. 4.17): 4–2; 4–1.
- Georgia—Whites (Fig. 4.18): 5–4; 5–3.
- California—Whites (Fig. 4.19): 4–1. Hispanics (Fig. 4.20): 4–1.

The disaggregated 5 States' data analysis showed the counties with the following greatest effect on COVID-19 deaths:

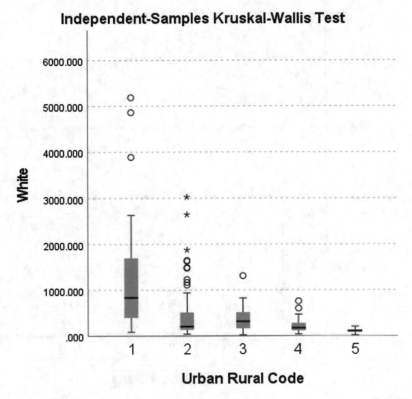

Fig. 4.6 COVID-19 deaths: Whites—14 States. (Source: CDC, 2021)

- The large fringe metro county among Whites; the large central metro among Blacks and Hispanics in New York.
- The large central metro for Whites, Blacks, and Hispanics in Texas.
- The large central metro among Whites; the large fringe metro among Blacks and Hispanics in Florida.
- The large central metro among Whites in Georgia.
- The large central metro among Whites and Hispanics in California.

Discussion

One research question in our exploratory empirical study was: were there differences in COVID-19 deaths among Whites, Blacks, and Hispanics across the urban-rural counties *nationwide*, in the *14 States*, and in the *5 States*? The data showed that there were statistically significant differences in median COVID-19 deaths overall among Whites, Blacks, and Hispanics across the six types of urban-rural counties

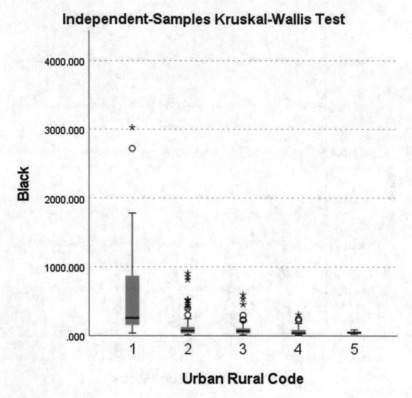

Fig. 4.7 COVID-19 deaths: Blacks—14 States. (Source: CDC, 2021)

nationwide, and in the 14 States. Disaggregating the nationwide and the 14 States' data by race/ethnicity also showed differences in COVID-19 deaths for each race/ ethnic group.

Data from the 5 States' showed differences in median COVID-19 deaths for each group of Whites, Blacks, and Hispanics among the six types of urban-rural counties in New York, Texas, and Florida; there were differences in the median COVID-19 deaths for Whites and Blacks in Georgia, and only for Whites and Hispanics in California among the urban-rural counties.

Another research question was: which counties had the strongest effect on COVID-19 deaths among Whites, Blacks, and Hispanics? The nationwide and the 14 States' data indicated that the large central metro county seemed to have the greatest impact on COVID-19 deaths overall among Whites, Blacks, and Hispanics. The disaggregated nationwide and 14 States' data analysis showed that the large fringe metro county had the greatest impact on COVID-19 deaths among Whites, and the large central metro with the strongest effect on COVID-19 deaths among Blacks and Hispanics.

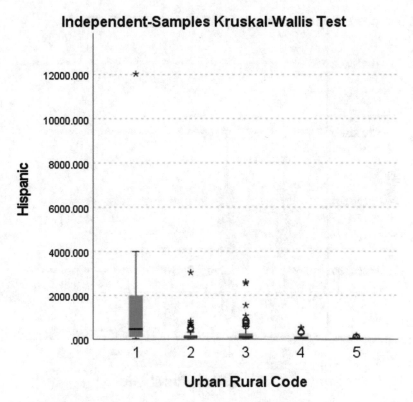

Fig. 4.8 COVID-19 deaths: Hispanics—14 States. (Source: CDC, 2021)

Table 4.4 Kruskal-Wallis Test summary—urban-rural counties (5 States)

States—urban-rural counties	Kruskal-Wallis H statistic		
	White	Black	Hispanic
New York	H (4) = 19.684, p < 0.001	H (3) = 14.230, p = 0.003	H (2) = 7.756, p = 0.021
Texas	H (4) = 24.733, p < 0.001	H (4) = 14.896, p = 0.005	H (4) = 23.927, p < 0.001
Florida	H (4) = 13.171, p = 0.010	H (4) =15.248, p = 0.004	H (3) = 14.644, p = 0.002
Georgia	H (4) = 18.448, p = 0.001	H (4) = 10.923, p = 0.027	H (4) = 2.745, p = 0.601
California	H (3) = 14.971, p = 0.002	H (2) =5.243, p = 0.073	H (3) =9.780, p = 0.021

Source: CDC (2021)

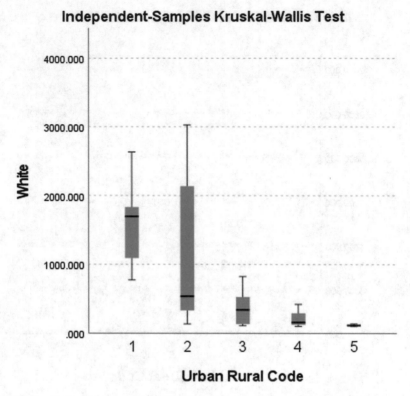

Fig. 4.9 New York—Whites. (Source: CDC, 2021)

The disaggregated 5 States' data showed the following counties in each of the 5 States with the most COVID-19 deaths: New York, large fringe metro (Whites) and large central metro (Blacks and Hispanics). Texas, large central metro (Whites, Blacks, and Hispanics). Florida, large central metro (Whites) and the large fringe metro (Blacks and Hispanics). Georgia, the large central metro (Whites). California, large central metro (Whites and Hispanics).

In addition to the analysis on the nationwide, 14 States and 5 States' data, we selected two of the top States of residence for Blacks (Florida and Georgia) to review their demographic overrepresentation in COVID-19 deaths. We looked at Alachua County, Clay County, and Leon County in Florida. In Georgia, counties with a high disproportionate representation in COVID-19 deaths among Blacks included Bulloch County, Coweta County, Fayette County, Fulton County, and Upson County. In relation to Florida, Blacks seemed to be demographically over-represented in COVID-19 deaths in counties with high poverty rates. Like Florida, Blacks in Georgia appeared to be disproportionately represented in COVID-19 deaths in counties with high poverty rates.

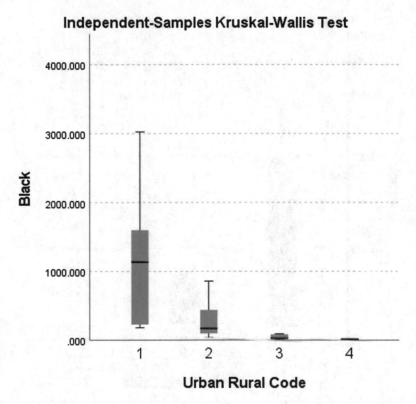

Fig. 4.10 New York—Blacks. (Source: CDC, 2021)

The findings in this study only on COVID-19 deaths among urban-rural counties would send a clear signal of some consistency with the general trend of a persisting demographic overrepresentation of Blacks and other people of color in COVID-19 cases, morbidity, hospitalizations, and deaths (Raine et al., 2020; Gu et al., 2020; Alcendor, 2020; Abedi et al., 2020; Kopel et al., 2020; Kim & Bostwick, 2020; Gross et al., 2020; Tartof et al., 2020; Moore et al., 2020; Rogers et al., 2020; Vahidy et al., 2020; Reed, 2021; Li et al., 2020; Kullar et al., 2020; Holtgrave et al., 2020; Mackey et al., 2020). However, that signal must now advance beyond rhetoric into some sort of bellwether phenomenon toward dismantling systemic racism.

Limitations of this exploratory empirical study included the unavailability of CDC data on COVID-19 deaths in counties with less than 100 deaths, which would more than likely be rural or semi-rural counties. Hence, the data we collected and used may have a potential urban bias. But we should note, too, that rural America is less racially and ethnically diverse than urban America (USDA, 2020); in 2018, the rural population comprised Whites (78.2%), Blacks (7.8%), and Hispanics (8.6%), and in 2018, urban America was populated with Whites (57.3%), Blacks (13.1%), and Hispanics (19.8%). In addition, the CDC dataset did not provide data on

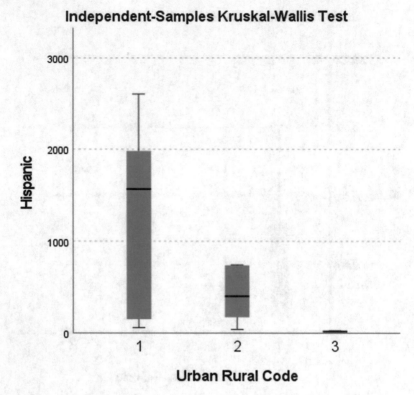

Fig. 4.11 New York—Hispanics. (Source: CDC, 2021)

COVID-19 deaths for many counties within the urban areas, where some urban counties were likely to have more than 100 deaths each; and the enormity of the sparse data is demonstrable, given that the CDC dataset covered a period of more than a year (from week-ending January 4, 2020 to April 17, 2021).

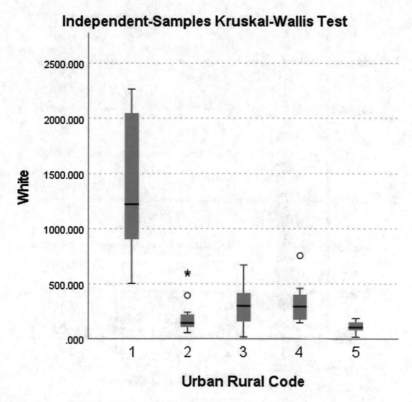

Fig. 4.12 Texas—Whites. (Source: CDC, 2021)

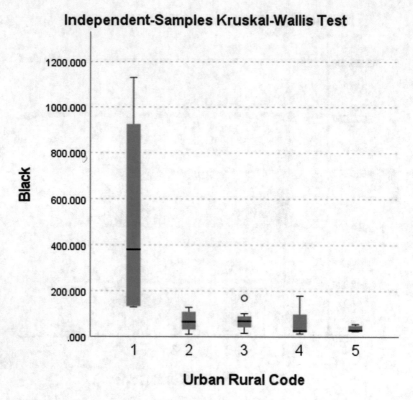

Fig. 4.13 Texas—Blacks. (Source: CDC, 2021)

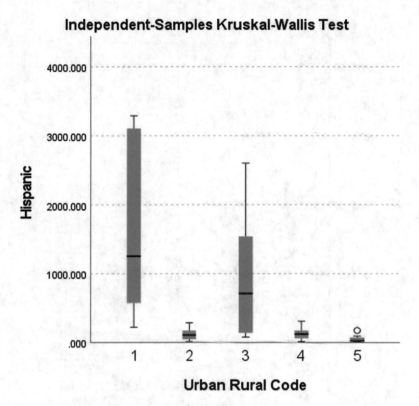

Fig. 4.14 Texas—Hispanics. (Source: CDC, 2021)

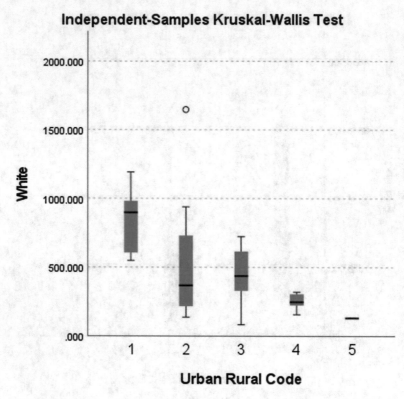

Fig. 4.15 Florida—Whites. (Source: CDC, 2021)

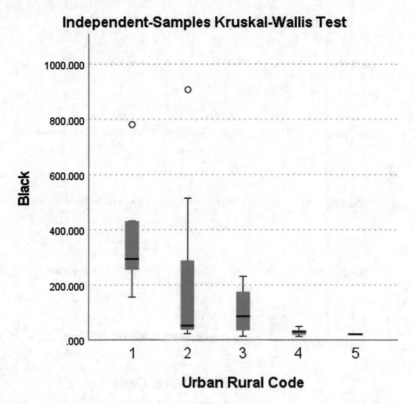

Fig. 4.16 Florida—Blacks. (Source: CDC, 2021)

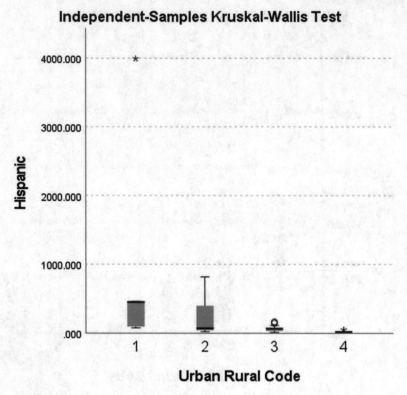

Fig. 4.17 Florida—Hispanics. (Source: CDC, 2021)

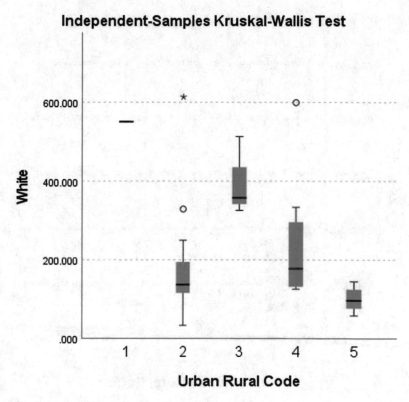

Fig. 4.18 Georgia—Whites. (Source: CDC, 2021)

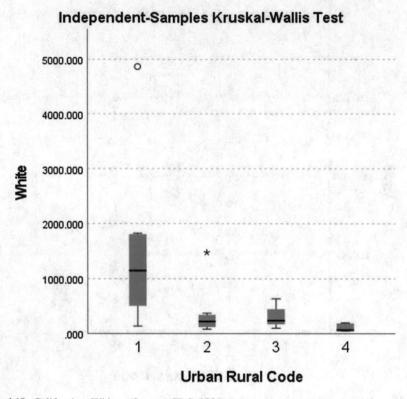

Fig. 4.19 California—Whites. (Source: CDC, 2021)

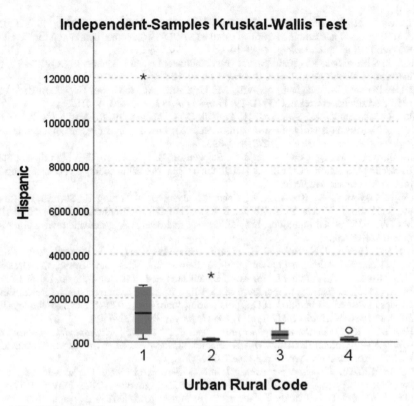

Fig. 4.20 California—Hispanics. (Source: CDC, 2021)

References

Abedi, V., Olulana, O., Avula, V., Chaudhary, D., Khan, A., Shahjouei, S., Li, J., & Zand, R. (2020). Racial, economic and health inequality and COVID-19 infection in the United States. *medRxiv*.

Alcendor, D. J. (2020). Racial disparities-associated COVID-19 mortality among minority populations in the US. *Journal of Clinical Medicine, 9*.

AP. (2020). Louisiana Data: Virus Hits Blacks, People With Hypertension. *U.S. News*, April 7, 2020.

CDC. (2021). *Provisional COVID-19 death counts by county and race* [Online]. CDC. Available: https://data.cdc.gov/NCHS/Provisional-COVID-19-Death-Counts-by-County-and-Ra/k8wy-p9cg/data. Accessed 14 Apr 2021.

Gross, C. P., Essien, U. R., Pasha, S., Gross, J. R., Wang, S. Y., & Nunez-Smith, M. (2020). Racial and ethnic disparities in population-level Covid-19 mortality. *Journal of General Internal Medicine, 35*, 3097–3099.

Gu, T., Mack, J. A., Salvatore, M., Prabhu Sankar, S., Valley, T. S., Singh, K., Nallamothu, B. K., Kheterpal, S., Lisabeth, L., Fritsche, L. G., & Mukherjee, B. (2020). Characteristics associated with racial/ethnic disparities in COVID-19 outcomes in an academic health care system. *JAMA Network Open, 3*, e2025197.

Holtgrave, D. R., Barranco, M. A., Tesoriero, J. M., Blog, D. S., & Rosenberg, E. S. (2020). Assessing racial and ethnic disparities using a COVID-19 outcomes continuum for New York State. *Annals of Epidemiology, 48*, 9–14.

Kim, S. J., & Bostwick, W. (2020). Social vulnerability and racial inequality in COVID-19 deaths in Chicago. *Health Education & Behavior, 47*, 509–513.

Kopel, J., Perisetti, A., Roghani, A., Aziz, M., Gajendran, M., & Goyal, H. (2020). Racial and gender-based differences in COVID-19. *Frontiers in Public Health, 8*, 418.

Kullar, R., Marcelin, J. R., Swartz, T. H., Piggott, D. A., Macias Gil, R., Mathew, T. A., & Tan, T. (2020). Racial disparity of coronavirus disease 2019 in African American communities. *The Journal of Infectious Diseases, 222*, 890–893.

Li, D., Gaynor, S. M., Quick, C., Chen, J. T., Stephenson, B. J. K., Coull, B. A., & Lin, X. (2020). Unraveling US national COVID-19 racial/ethnic disparities using county level data among 328 million Americans. *medRxiv*.

Mackey, K., Ayers, C. K., Kondo, K. K., Saha, S., Advani, S. M., Young, S., Spencer, H., Rusek, M., Anderson, J., Veazie, S., Smith, M., & Kansagara, D. (2020). Racial and ethnic disparities in COVID-19-related infections, hospitalizations, and deaths: A systematic review. *Annals of Internal Medicine*.

Moore, J. T., Ricaldi, J. N., Rose, C. E., Fuld, J., Parise, M., Kang, G. J., Driscoll, A. K., Norris, T., Wilson, N., Rainisch, G., Valverde, E., Beresovsky, V., Agnew Brune, C., Oussayef, N. L., Rose, D. A., Adams, L. E., Awel, S., Villanueva, J., Meaney-Delman, D., & Honein, M. A. (2020). Disparities in Incidence of COVID-19 Among Underrepresented Racial/Ethnic Groups in Counties Identified as Hotspots During June 5–18, 2020–22 States, February–June 2020. *MMWR. Morbidity and Mortality Weekly Report, 69*, 1122–1126.

NCHS/CDC. (2021). *Health disparities provisional death counts for coronavirus disease 2019 (COVID-19)* [Online]. NCHS, CDC. Available: https://www.cdc.gov/nchs/nvss/vsrr/covid19/health_disparities.htm. Accessed 5 June 2021.

NYSDOH. (2020). *Fatalities by county* [Online]. New York State Department of Health. Available: https://covid19tracker.health.ny.gov/views/NYS-COVID19-Tracker/NYSDOHCOVID-19Tracker-Fatalities?%3Aembed=yes&%3Atoolbar=no&%3Atabs=n. Accessed 1 May 2021.

Raine, S., Liu, A., Mintz, J., Wahood, W., Huntley, K., & Haffizulla, F. (2020). Racial and ethnic disparities in COVID-19 outcomes: Social determination of health. *International Journal of Environmental Research and Public Health, 17*.

Reed, D. D. (2021). Racial disparities in healthcare: How COVID-19 ravaged one of the wealthiest African American counties in the United States. *Social Work in Public Health, 36*, 118–127.

Reyes, C., Husain, N., Gutowski, C., Clair, S. S., & Pratt, G. (2020). Chicago's coronavirus disparity: Black Chicagoans are dying at nearly six times the rate of white residents, data show. *Chicago Tribune, 7*, 2020.

Rogers, T. N., Rogers, C. R., Vansant-Webb, E., Gu, L. Y., Yan, B. & Qeadan, F. 2020. Racial disparities in COVID-19 mortality among essential Workers in the United States. World Med Health Policy.

Rossen, L. M., Branum, A. M., Ahmad, F. B., Sutton, P., & Anderson, R. N. (2020). Excess deaths associated with COVID-19, by age and race and ethnicity - United States, January 26-October 3, 2020. *MMWR. Morbidity and Mortality Weekly Report, 69*, 1522–1527.

Tartof, S. Y., Qian, L., Hong, V., Wei, R., Nadjafi, R. F., Fischer, H., Li, Z., Shaw, S. F., Caparosa, S. L., Nau, C. L., Saxena, T., Rieg, G. K., Ackerson, B. K., Sharp, A. L., Skarbinski, J., Naik, T. K., & Murali, S. B. (2020). Obesity and mortality among patients diagnosed with COVID-19: Results from an integrated health care organization. *Annals of Internal Medicine, 173*, 773–781.

Thebault, R., Tran, A. B. & Williams, V. 2020. *The coronavirus is infecting and killing black Americans at an alarmingly high rate* [Online]. The Washington Post. Available: https://www.washingtonpost.com/nation/2020/04/07/coronavirus-is-infecting-killing-black-americans-an-alarmingly-high-rate-post-analysis-shows/?arc404=true. Accessed 12 July 2020.

USCB. (2019). *QuickFacts United States* [Online]. United States Census Bureau. Available: https://www.census.gov/quickfacts/fact/table/US/RHI125219. Accessed 18 May 2021.

USDA. (2020). *Racial and ethnic minorities made up about 22 percent of the rural population in 2018, compared to 43 percent in urban areas* [Online]. USDA. Available: https://www. ers.usda.gov/data-products/chart-gallery/gallery/chart-detail/?chartId=99538. Accessed 10 Aug 2021.

Vahidy, F. S., Nicolas, J. C., Meeks, J. R., Khan, O., Pan, A., Jones, S. L., Masud, F., Sostman, H. D., Phillips, R., Andrieni, J. D., Kash, B. A., & Nasir, K. (2020). Racial and ethnic dispari-ties in SARS-CoV-2 pandemic: Analysis of a COVID-19 observational registry for a diverse US metropolitan population. *BMJ Open, 10*, e039849.

Wortham, J. M., Lee, J. T., Althomsons, S., Latash, J., Davidson, A., Guerra, K. & Murray, K. (2020). *Characteristics of persons who died with COVID-19 — United States, February 12–May 18, 2020* [Online]. Atlanta, GA: MMWR, CDC. Available: https://doi.org/10.15585/mmwr.mm6928e1externalicon. Accessed 25 Mar 2021.

Yancy, C. W. (2020). COVID-19 and African Americans. *JAMA, 323*(19), 1891–1892. https://doi.org/10.1001/jama.2020.6548

Chapter 5
Dismantling Systemic Racism and Structuration Theory

This book commences in Chap. 1 with a focus on racial health disparities and segregated health care in America alongside poor health outcomes experienced by the racially disadvantaged people of color, amid rising health expenditures as a percentage of gross domestic product (GDP). We then turned to epidemiology to present the beginnings of COVID-19 in Chap. 2; to explain the characteristics of this highly infectious virus, as a percent of asymptomatic infections, infection fatality ratio, case fatality rate, reproduction number, incubation period, latent period, and serial interval; to provide data on the COVID-19 devastation experienced by people of color; and a note on the mishandling of the pandemic. Chapter 3 outlines a brief historic overview of White-imposed racism as part of the structural foundation of colonial America and examines Feagin's systemic racism that operates through the White racial frame, and Eduardo Bonilla-Silva's racialized social systems, racial hierarchy, and the allocation of rewards within the structure of color-blind racism. Furthermore, Chap. 3 advances a research proposal to study the role of spatial differences (urban-rural classification) on COVID-19 deaths among Whites, Blacks, and Hispanics in the 50 States and DC. Chapter 4 presents the results of this study, utilizing primarily the CDC dataset (January 1, 2020–April, 17, 2021) on Provisional COVID-19 Deaths by County, and Race and Hispanic Origin, with the existing data from 760 counties within 50 States and DC (CDC, 2021). Apparently, there have been numerous studies on racial health disparities, with minimal impact on disparities, prompting this conclusion: for more than 50 years, health researchers have been focusing on health disparities, but disparities are still reigning supreme; so dismantling systemic racism as a pathway toward racial equity becomes critical; hence, health researchers should change their focus on health disparities toward a focus on the core causes of systemic racism (Lavizzo-Mourey et al., 2021). Hence, Chap. 5 analyzes the link between duality of structure in structuration theory with the White racial frame as the platform, in its search for theoretical pathways toward dismantling systemic racism.

© The Author(s), under exclusive license to Springer Nature
Switzerland AG 2022
P. Misir, *COVID-19 and Health System Segregation in the US*, Springer Briefs
in Public Health, https://doi.org/10.1007/978-3-030-88766-7_5

The dramatic and disproportionate COVID-19 devastation foisted on the working poor people of color in the USA in itself warrants publishing to a global audience. The intent of this book was not merely to shine the spotlight on the link between systemic racism as a fundamental cause of poor health and racial health disparities, but to identify strategies that would end racism. The COVID-19 devastation inflicted on the historically disadvantaged minorities within the racialized and segregated health-care system is not a novel phenomenon. The constant drumbeat of long-standing systemic health and social inequities placing Blacks and other disadvantaged people at high risk of exposure and infection with COVID-19 has been a pulsating repetitious sound that surfaces at every disease outbreak/epidemic or other natural disasters. Besides, amid COVID-19, many Blacks and other racial minorities have long transcended this "high-risk stage," as many have already died, without even a pittance done to demolish health disparities and the race and class-based segregated health care. Racial health disparities stem from social conditions, not from racial features, deeply grounded in systemic racism, which operates through the White racial frame to dominate racially disadvantaged and marginalized people of color in the USA.

History is replete with accounts of marginalized groups as the enemies of pandemics and other disasters, which have invariably trailed "the international fault lines of inequality, poverty, and neglect" (Snowden, 2019 p. 38). But what are the origins of inequality, poverty, and neglect? Granted that a pandemic can unleash its fury and destroy the way of life of people, exponentially increasing inequality, poverty, and neglect. But political domination has been more of a constant than pandemics in sustaining inequality, poverty, and neglect and also constructing and reconstructing social stratification in society. In the USA, the genesis of racial marginalization and social deprivation as outcomes of White domination and the White racial frame against Blacks reverts to the year 1619. Clearly then, if domination against Blacks had its origins in 1619, then the current upsurge of so many repetitious findings and information on racial health disparities are not novel, as evidence has been accruing long before the emergence of the COVID-19 pandemic, and at least way back to the Jamestown Settlement in 1619.

Since the White settlement at Jamestown in 1619, provision of health care for Blacks was never a priority, especially for poor Blacks, whose only choice was to claim their dubious space as reluctant victims to poor health for 400 years and counting. People in the USA would agree that there has been much progress in health-care expenditures, medicine, public health, and medical technology. Yet alongside such advancement remains the institutionalized race and class-based segregation of health care, leading to the inevitable and seemingly permanent Black health crisis (Byrd & Clayton, 2012), characterized by persistent segregation of the race and class-based health system; the crisis is a continuation of race and class-based structural health inequalities and inequities and long-lasting underrepresentation of Blacks in medicine and public health. Even though the Civil Rights Act of 1964 and Medicare in 1965 viewed race and class-based segregation of health care as illegal, de facto race and class-based segregation of health-care systems has remained unfettered, principally due to the residential segregation of Blacks. The

US health system operates on the doctrine of "separate but equal," whereby the dominant group has access to quality health care and the people of color have access to a lesser or zero health care. The "separation" implies and enforces inferiority in health care for people of color. Thus, it was hardly surprising then that despite the huge US national health expenditures, for example, 21.3% of GDP in 2020, key poor health outcomes within a race and class-based segregated health-care system persist around infant mortality, life expectancy, maternal mortality, mortality, cancer, cardiovascular health, women's health, HIV/AIDS, and, indeed, the ever-present COVID-19. Hence, racial institutionalization of poor health outcomes further progresses racial health disparities.

In relation to the current pandemic, several studies, among others (Raine et al., 2020; Gu et al., 2020; Alcendor, 2020; Abedi et al., 2020; Kopel et al., 2020; Kim & Bostwick, 2020; Gross et al., 2020; Tartof et al., 2020; Moore et al., 2020; Rogers et al., 2020; Vahidy et al., 2020; Reed, 2021; Li et al., 2020; Kullar et al., 2020; Holtgrave et al., 2020), have demonstrated the overrepresentation of the racially disadvantaged and marginalized people of color in COVID-19 cases, morbidity, hospitalizations, and deaths. These researchers have performed yeoman service in highlighting the highly contagious and racialized trajectory of COVID-19 mortality. Hence, "People of color are dying disproportionally from COVID-19… as a result of our racialized social system" (Bonilla-Silva, 2020, p. 7).

Even amid COVID-19, the evidence on racial health disparities experienced by Blacks and other people of color in the country is overwhelming, but that vast evidence has been staring at Americans for countless years now! The concept of racial health disparities is not a new phenomenon. But every time a new pandemic or disaster comes to town, we regurgitate the same stories of Blacks and other historically racially disadvantaged groups' demographic overrepresentation in cases, hospitalizations, and deaths. Then the pandemic/disaster subsequently dissipates, but racial health disparities live to reign supreme for another day. The Institute of Medicine Report on *Unequal Treatment: Confronting Racial and Ethnic Disparities in Health Care* concluded in 2002 "that the real challenge lies not in debating whether disparities exist, because the evidence is overwhelming, but in the developing and implementing of strategies to reduce and eliminate them" (Nelson, 2002 p. 667).

Without a doubt, there is overpowering evidence of racial health disparities experienced by Blacks and other racially disadvantaged groups. But identifying their cause has attracted persisting disagreements, with claims that racial health disparities are initiated by race-based genetic difference or race-neutral economic difference. Nevertheless, both justifications were debunked, as they overlooked the roots of health disparities in social inequality (Roberts, 2012). The cultural persistence of race and racism has remained a long-lasting motif of American society (Du Bois, 2007; Myrdal, 1962; Hacker, 2010), where systemic racism and racial oppression operating through the White racial frame were important ingredients in the structural foundation of colonial America and its racialized social systems and have even endured as a US foundation (Feagin, 2020). However, COVID-19 has now brought racial health disparities against Blacks and other disadvantaged groups of color into even sharper focus, showing that racism in health care and public health institutions has now become transformed into a robust social, moral, and human crisis, where its resolution demands more than rhetoric. How do we bring an end to these persistent racial health disparities emanating from systemic racism?

In Pursuit of Systemic Solutions

For 400 years and counting, Blacks and, subsequently, other historically racially disadvantaged populations in the USA have been facing persisting health disparities in the use of preventive and other health services. There is no question that a strong sense of our racial past would offer a better sense of the racial present, showing that racial oppression in the form of genocide against the American Indian, Black enslavement, legal segregation, and White-imposed racism was embedded in the foundational reality of colonial America (Feagin, 2020). Any crusade with a strategy to reduce or eliminate racial health disparities may be doomed to failure, if that strategy primarily focuses on the disparities and does not recognize the fact that the foundation of American society is rotten to the core with systemic racism.

That said, the dominant power holders have always found replaceable mechanisms to modulate the impact of any intervention aimed at reducing disparities. A systematic review (Nelson et al., 2020) of 125 articles over the period January 1, 1996, through July 5, 2019, studied the effects of barriers generating health disparities in 10 preventive services for adults and to assess the efficacy of interventions to lessen the disparities. It found inadequate or low strength of evidence and applicability for most interventions, which demonstrated difficulties for achieving health equity and reducing racial health disparities for Blacks and other people of color. Not surprisingly, a recent study found that:

> Over the past half-century, understanding of health and health care disparities in the United States — including underlying social, clinical, and system-level contributors — has increased. Yet disparities persist. Eliminating health disparities will require a movement away from disparities as the focus of research and toward a research agenda centered on achieving racial equity by dismantling structural racism. (Lavizzo-Mourey et al., 2021, p. 1681)

Racial health disparities are growing as well as the number of studies on disparities, as can be observed amid COVID-19. This pandemic has attracted an outbreak of studies to underscore the disproportionality in morbidity and mortality among racial/ethnic minorities and other vulnerable populations compared to Whites. How many of these studies perceive systemic racism as a primary factor inducing the persistence of racial health disparities? However, many similar studies predating COVID-19 were disengaged from the context of institutionalized racial oppression (Hardeman, 2020). In fact, a meta-analysis of 293 articles showed that racism was significantly correlated with poorer mental and physical health (Paradies et al., 2015). Nonetheless, many articles in attempting to explain the factors associated with physical and mental well-being have not used the concepts of structural racism/systemic racism.

For instance, a predominant feature in a systematic review of 85 articles (Castle et al., 2019) was non-use of the term *racism* or not naming *systemic racism* as the foundation of health outcome disparities. Some 16 out of 25 articles used the term *institutionalized racism*, from which only 4 were original research papers (Hardeman et al., 2018). In its 39-year history, the *Health Affairs* journal mentioned racism only in 114 papers (Boyd et al., 2020). *The Lancet* journal revealed that most articles that mentioned *race* did not also mention *structural racism* and *systemic racism* (Bailey et al., 2017). Then a PubMed database search showed that only 86 articles contained the terms *race, institutional racism*, and *structural racism* (Cullen et al., 2020). From one health crisis to the next, and COVID-19 is not novel in this regard, we see the same story line with studies underlining racial health disparities.

Understanding racism eclectically involves seeing racism as multidimensional and systemic, extending beyond racial bias (Feagin & Bennefield, 2014), a link between racist ideologies and racist structures (Golash-Boza, 2016), as systemic and embedded in differences in power between the races, and the racialized social system method (Bonilla-Silva, 2015), and intersectionality, where the power relations of race, class, and gender input each other and work collectively (Collins & Bilge, 2020). Crenshaw (1989), in a trailblazing paper, exposes the failure of laws to alleviate discrimination, due to a dependence on a "single axis framework" of law that proffers a feeble analysis resolution, when the issues intersect. Further, understanding racism necessitates a recognition that structural gendered racism is the holistic link between structural racism and structural sexism in influencing race and gender inequities. Thus, while applying an intersectional analysis, structural gendered racism is exposed as a root cause of health problems among women of color, essentially reducing the risk of COVID-19 troubles (Laster Pirtle & Wright, 2021). Nevertheless, applying intersectionality of issues as the link between gender, race, and class in population health could be influenced by the White racial frame and systemic racism.

Studies have found that individuals who related experiencing racism unveil worse health than people who did not relate such experiences (Williams & Mohammed, 2009). While this approach had been vital in moving the conversation from innate differences in biology or culture to social exposures, it was insufficient because of its sparse attention to the multiple dimensions of racism, and especially structural racism (Gee & Ford, 2011). However, Williams and Mohammed in their study acknowledged the need for a multidimensional approach to dismantle racism, thus: "Moreover, there is substantial progress yet to be made in dismantling the institutional structures, processes, and policies that undergird societal racism" (Williams & Mohammed, 2009, p. 40). Possibly, an understanding of structural racism as it pertains to individual and population health is still at the embryonic stage (Bailey et al., 2017; Williams & Mohammed, 2013).

Understanding racism would signal that a large proportion of White Americans has, at all times, been White nationalists, supporting White supremacy, using extreme versions of the White racial frame to spout openly and aggressively White nationalist, supremacist ideas, according to Feagin in an interview with The Sociologist; he argued that this supremacist posturing represents the White resistance to the browning of America, as the White population becomes lesser each year (The Sociologist, 2020).

Understanding racism requires an acknowledgement of the active role of politics and a political will to confront racial oppression. Any sustainable racism is rooted in politics that facilitates the reproduction of racial domination. In the fight against racism, we should also acknowledge Richard Wright's assertion in 1946 about America, "There isn't any Negro problem; there is only a white problem. The problem is white because only whites can resolve it. Whites number 130,000,000 compared to 15,000,000 blacks. They hold the political, industrial, and social power. They are everything…The problem is a white problem because it is the whites who pose it every day" (Kinnamon & Fabre, 1993, p. 99). However, Whites have had 400 years to bring closure to racial oppression, which still it continues to stalk the land and its institutions with persisting health inequalities and inequities.

Blacks and other poor racial minorities, so trapped in brutality, marginalization, and deprivation, can paint a revealing picture of poverty and vulnerability and how they are being distributed. But even the image and contours of poverty and vulnerability can be shaped and reshaped through the ruling scientific perspective of the day, especially given that poverty and vulnerability are fundamental to risk exposure and outcomes of COVID-19. For instance, influenced by the logic that multiple mechanisms can contribute to a persistent relationship between a cause and an effect (Lieberson, 1987) and a persistent relationship between SES and disease (House et al., 1990), Link and Phelan (1995) formulated their theory of SES as a fundamental cause of health inequalities.

However, in a later study (Phelan & Link, 2015), they posited that health inequalities arising from fundamental causes would not be eliminated through intervention mechanisms, since persistent inequalities in knowledge, money, power, prestige, etc., make certain that such intervention mechanisms are replaceable. They then qualified the relationship between SES and racial health inequalities as "We conclude that the connection between race and health outcomes endures largely because racism is a fundamental cause of racial differences in SES and because SES is a fundamental cause of health inequalities, but that racism also has a fundamental association with health outcomes independent of SES" (Phelan & Link, 2015 p. 325). To lay bare the partial potency of SES, a study of 26 million beneficiaries of Medicare in 1993 showed that while race and income had effects, race was the predominant determinant of racial health disparities in care and even adjustment for income hardly altered the racial health disparities between Blacks and Whites (Geiger, 1996).

Understanding 'racism' requires both a moral and an explanatory conception; 'racism' as a moral concept is an expression of moral condemnation, and as an explanatory concept, it is an expression of illuminating social problems that systematically harm non-Whites (Cabezas, 2021). But in his book, *Re-Defining Racism: A Philosophical Analysis*, Alberto Urquidez (2020) explained that there is an unremitting need to probe this concept of racism, hotly contested, as the concept is not only intellectual but politicized and emotionally charged as well, confirming its significance. As so much harangue is entangled with the nature of racism, Urquidez proposed an essential methodological clarification to the question "What is racism?" a sort of investigation into the concept of racism, in order to reach a consensus through developing a moral theory of racism. Perhaps, any dismantling of systemic racism would require a working consensus on the meaning of racism because of its multiple competing sociological perspectives.

Urquidez sees the moral theory of racism as referring to phenomena sustaining racial oppression, the core of racism, and attributions of racism are justified, where they contribute to sustaining racial oppression. Racism should be the subject of constant moral condemnation as a result of the systematic harms it inflicts on subordinate racial groups. But he contended that racism is not merely about addressing personal harms, since it positions racial oppression, that is, White supremacy, in structure, upholding racially differential treatment, where the victimized non-Whites are reduced to a condition of vulnerability.

Urquidez (2020) noted that racism is racial oppression that has an affinity with White supremacy's lexes: racial slavery, racial segregation, and racial apartheid, along with the new forms of racism, such as race-neutral and color-blind racism. In order to progress this consensus on the concept of racism, Urquidez explained that the frame of the victimized racial group must not only address personal morality with a focus on individual responsibility and blame but also on political morality, with a focus on injustice and oppression. Perhaps, a strategy for dismantling racism may demand a focus on a blended mix of individual, interpersonal, and systemic racism.

Understanding racism requires exposing these characteristics: the mechanisms and practices (behaviors, styles, cultural affectations, traditions, and organizational procedures) at the social, economic, ideological, and political levels, which are involved in the reproduction of racial domination (Bonilla-Silva, 2015); the racialized social systems (refer to Chap. 3 for an explanation) within "societies in which economic, political, social, and ideological levels are partially structured by the placement of actors in racial categories or races" (Bonilla-Silva, 2001, p.37), with a changing racial hierarchy, comprising races at different levels creating racial contestation; such racialized social systems differentially distribute rewards to racial groups along racial lines (Bonilla-Silva, 1997); both positive and negative racial attitudes are linked to racial ideology (Golash-Boza, 2016); Jim Crow racism was the glue for championing a ruthless and overt system of racial oppression in the pre-Civil Rights era; and color-blind racism today is the ideological protection for a covert and institutionalized system in the post-Civil Rights era (Bonilla-Silva, 2013). Understanding racism requires a recognition that its most important effects are structural or institutional and do not need intent, as is necessary, at the individual level (Bonilla-Silva, 2020). In fact, the most relevant grounds for legal redress on racial health discrimination is a focus on effect (Watson, 1994), not intent, meaning that the focus on effect underscores group and not individual outcomes of racial oppression (King, 1996).

It is common knowledge now that the marginalized and racially disadvantaged people of color are the most vulnerable and susceptible to pandemics and other disasters and in their after-effects. Blacks and Hispanics have been demographically overrepresented in COVID-19 deaths, which have occurred due to the racialized social systems (Bonilla-Silva, 1997), but more so because of color-blind racism, where structural racism becomes minimized. Bonilla-Silva (2020, p. 2) explained that:

> …color-blind racial framing…limits recognizing that the problems made apparent during the COVID-19 pandemic have a structural nature (e.g., class and racial inequalities, the lack of a proper safety net, and the need for universal health care). More significantly for my analysis, structural racism is mostly dislodged (or minimized) as a central factor shaping the nation.

He pointed out that the core of color-blind racism is to describe racial scenarios as nonracial, enabling more individualized action on culture or biology, with lesser emphasis on the structural causes of inequalities. Hence, with the progression of active color-blind racism, it is likely that the White racial frame has experienced a metamorphosis from being overt, as it were during Jim Crow, to becoming covert within racialized social systems in the post-Civil Rights era.

Other recommendations for clinicians and researchers to dismantle structural racism include, inter alia, understanding the historical roots of racial health disparities (Hardeman et al., 2016; Bailey et al., 2021). Clearly, facilitating an understanding of the roots of health disparities, inter alia, inclusive of cross-cultural training and education and their derivatives (anti-racism training, diversity training, cultural competence, cultural safety, cultural humility, cultural intelligence) for clinicians and other health-care professionals, is a laudable pursuit; but these programs have been a common activity in the USA following the Civil Rights legislation in the 1960s (Anand & Winters, 2008); and not long after, focusing on health workforce cultural competence became a common approach to progressing health service quality for culturally and ethnically diverse groups, resulting in concerns on evidence strength and quality (Jongen et al., 2018). In concluding remarks on the nature of such training programs, Shepherd (2019, p. 8) had this to say:

> Cultural awareness workshops and their derivatives are often well-intentioned…Yet these interventions are implemented without evidence and exist on face validity alone. Decades of research point to their ineffectiveness, despite billions of dollars being spent on their operation. Workshop approaches are often over-generalizing, simplistic and impractical. Broader expectations of reductions in health disparities are almost certainly unachievable.

In the quest to end racism, Guess (2006) argued that sociological scholarship of racism in America characteristically has focused on Blacks. So there is little understanding of how Whites sustain White privilege. The fact that people are living and interacting in a White supremacist world would require a better understanding of Whiteness, in order to overcome racism (Bonilla-Silva, 2015). Ferber's (1998, p. 60) concept of White identity and its relationship to White supremacy also reinforces the view for a better understanding of White identity:

> …we cannot comprehend white supremacist racism without exploring the construction of white identity. White identity defines itself in opposition to inferior others; racism, then, becomes the maintenance of white identity . . . When researchers fail to explore the construction of 'race', they contribute to the reproduction of 'race' as a naturally existing category.

Guess (2006) also noted that Omi and Winant (1986), Roediger (1999), Feagin (2001), West (1994), Frankenburg (1993), and Ignatiev and Garvey (1996) were only a small number of people, who have been promoting antiracist scholarship and the social construction of whiteness. West (2002, p. 47), perhaps gaining the nod from this small group of scholars, voiced strong language on the plight of Blacks:

> The notion that black people are human beings is a relatively new discovery in the modern West. The idea of black equality in beauty, culture, and intellectual capacity remains problematic and controversial within prestigious halls of learning and sophisticated intellectual circles. The Afro-American encounter with the modern world has been shaped first and foremost by the doctrine of white supremacy, which is embodied in institutional practices and enacted in everyday folkways under varying circumstances and evolving conditions.

Apparently, West's position is that America's race problem is a White problem, and its resolution mandates a focus on White supremacy. Richard Wright also voiced a similar view, that America's problem is White!

Hence, Guess (2006) explained that in order to review both sides of the Black and White binary paradigm of race, it is critical to understand its structuration. This brings us to Giddens' work on structuration theory (Giddens, 1984), where the focus is on the agents' (human subjects) activities/social practices.

Structuration Theory: Agency and Structure

According to Giddens (1979), the theory of structuration was born because there was no theory of action in the social sciences; functionalism and structuralism, by failing to depict action as a constant flow through time and space, generated the dualisms of individual/society, subject/object, and conscious/unconscious modes of cognition, resulting in no link between agency and structure; together, these dualisms have undermined the growth of a theory of action; hence, the theory of structuration was aimed at integrating agency and structure to constitute a duality. In this sense, structure cannot exist without agency and agency (agents as human subjects) cannot exist without structure (rules and resources); human action requires structure, and structure requires human action, and agency and structure are interlinked in constant and recursive human action or practice (Ritzer, 2011).

Fundamental to sustaining the integration between agency and structure in society is the agents' (people, human subjects) knowledge, arising from three layers of consciousness and action (Giddens, 1984): (1) reflexive monitoring of action (agents monitor their own activities and expect others to do the same, along with monitoring their social and physical contexts) and discursive consciousness (where people have the capacity to describe the conditions of their actions in words); (2) rationalizations of actions (where people seek security by rationalizing their social life through developing routines or habitual activities) and practical consciousness (where people implicitly have the knowledge about what they do and the reasons for doing what they do, but they do not verbalize this knowledge); and (3) motivation for action (wants and desires) and unconscious motives/cognition (where people may suppress their semiotic desires). All three systems of action and consciousness are involved in the production and reproduction of social systems.

The conceptual essentials of structuration theory hinges on structure, system, and duality of structure (Giddens, 1984); thus, structure refers to rules and resources and does not exist in time and space, but only through the actions of agents, and structure is both constraining and enabling for human action; social systems are reproduced human practices, usually the unanticipated consequences of agents' activities, and take on structural properties, and the idea of the duality of structure is that "…the structural properties of social systems are both medium and outcome of the practices they recursively organize" (Giddens, 1984, p. 25).

The Duality of Structure: White Racial Frame

Giddens (1984) introduces the dimensions of the duality of structure as structure (social systems), modality, and interaction:

(Structural properties)	Signification	Domination	Legitimation
(Modality)	Interpretive schemes	Facilities	Norm
(Interaction)	Communication	Power	Sanction

We will now theoretically show how the duality of structure impacts systemic racism that operates through the White racial frame, racialized social systems, and color-blind racism. Relating to this duality of structure, agents (White racists) produce/reproduce three dimensions of interaction: communication, power, and sanction by drawing on three corresponding complementary dimensions of structure; rules of signification (involving use of language, e.g., cognition in the White racial frame and racialized social systems, as racially framed interpretations and narratives; resources of domination); allocative (involving control of materials, e.g., as cutting back government programs largely benefiting communities of color, underfunded racial health disparities research at National Institutes of Health (NIH)) or authoritative (involving control of people, e.g., powerful health-related White decision makers' control of communities of color in all major institutions); and rules of legitimation (involving moral rules governing appropriate behavior, e.g., morally rationalizing the White racial frame and racialized social systems through color-blind racism). Agents access structures to produce/reproduce interactions/practices vis-à-vis modalities. The modality of interpretive scheme (e.g., cognitive knowledge of the White racial frame and racialized social systems relating to language/nonverbal codes) links signification structures with the interaction dimension of communication. The modality of facility (e.g., capacity to sustain the White racial frame and racialized social systems via authoritative and allocative control) links domination structures with exercising power in interaction. The norm modality (e.g., beliefs, values, policies, procedures pertaining to the White racial frame and racialized social systems) links legitimation structures with the sanctioning of communities of color in interaction.

The Duality of Structure: The Black Resistance

Applying structuration theory to the Black resistance demonstrates a recursive interchange of Black resistance between the dimensions of structure, the dimensions of interaction, and their corresponding modalities, with illustrations largely from the Black Lives Matter (BLM) movement (Nummi et al., 2019). The Black resistance agents produce/reproduce three dimensions of interaction for Black counter-framing against the White racial frame and racialized social systems: communication, power, and sanction by drawing on three corresponding complementary dimensions of structure (rules of signification, resources of domination, and rules of legitimation):

- Rules of signification (involving use of cognitive language and coding that call for dismantling of the White racial frame and racialized social systems as a racial ideology for racial equality, racial justice, and real police reform).
- Resources of domination: allocative (involving increasing and effective use of social media platforms; use of the #BlackLivesMatter (BLM) hashtag; use of alternative Black media; participation in social movement via users' cell phones, tablets, and laptops; the phenomenon of Black Twitter; sharing street and other photos of peaceful protesters, of young black gang members shielding a store from being looted, and of young black men in post-protest cleaning up; petitions on police abuses and the George Floyd Justice in Policing Act of 2021) or authoritative (involving a relationship with Black social media users, a key black counterpublic, Black women as targets for the police, BLM Chapters, developing trainees).
- Rules of legitimation (involving moral rules to end racist behavior through morally counter-framing the White racial frame, racialized social systems and color-blind racism, heteronormativity, emphasis on Black women and LGBTQ people).

Black resistance agents create and recreate interactions/social practices vis-à-vis modalities. The modality of interpretive scheme (e.g., cognitive knowledge to end racism through language/nonverbal codes) links signification structures with the interaction dimension of communication. The modality of facility (e.g., capacity and capability to end systemic racial oppression via authoritative and allocative control) connects domination structures with exercising power in interaction. The norm modality (e.g., beliefs, values, policies, procedures pertaining to ending racial oppression) links legitimation structures with the sanctioning of upholders of the White racial frame, racialized social systems, and color-blind racism.

Structuration Theory Informing the Chauvin Case

A powerful example of the White racial frame and the Black resistance counter-frame, and indeed, the racial dialectic, can be observed in a discussion of the Derek Chauvin verdict in Minnesota, and Black and White perspectives on policing racism with Stanford University scholars Hakeem Jefferson, Robert Weisberg, and Matthew Clair (Witte & Driscoll, 2021). An example of use of the White racial frame would be court cases involving the police, where prosecutors traditionally have conceded to police officers' testimony on the reasonableness of their application of force and would not prosecute on those grounds, as in the 2014 case of the St. Louis Prosecuting Attorney refusing to indict the White police officer Darren Wilson for the murder of the Black teenager Michael Brown.

The Chauvin case was different, in that the world and the jurors saw Chauvin's knee on George Floyd's neck for 9 min and 29 s, whereby prosecutors addressed the unreasonableness of Chauvin's application of force and deemed him a rogue police officer (Witte & Driscoll, 2021), setting in motion counter-framing as a contrast or counter to the White racial frame. The counter-frame produced a different prosecutorial approach, a deviation from the norm, which went through the process of deframing. Through deframing, prosecutors reframed the concept of Chauvin as culpable without besmirching policing as an institution, by demonstrating the glaring unambiguity of the Floyd killing, and enabling the jurors to perceive Chauvin as guilty. Reframing may deliver these new perspectives as test cases for policing policing, thus: a different prosecutorial approach with the State Attorney General rather than the local prosecutor taking the lead; a focus on judges questioning police practices and issuing warrants; and accountability for police officers, as they hardly become indicted for murder or manslaughter, in allegations of excess usage of police force as well as other police abuses.

Clearly, the Black resistance counter-framing and deframing activities impacted the Chauvin case, simultaneously highlighting the significance of "agents" and "agency." Apparently, the Attorney General as an agent, through its lead in the Chauvin case, facilitated greater allocative and authoritative resources of domination to the prosecutors as agents in the execution of their responsibilities. The fact that the Attorney General took the lead and not the local prosecutor, as is usually the case, symbolized the exercise of power to establish greater diligence than in the past on allegations of police violence against communities of color and, perhaps, to bring an end to the preexisting state of affairs on allegations against the police; in the past, prosecutors accepted the police testimony, and so would not prosecute. Following Giddens (1984), agents, by definition, have the capability and knowledge to make a difference. It was quite likely that notwithstanding the Black resistance impact on the Chauvin case, these agents (Attorney General and prosecutors) employed counter-framing, encompassing deframing and reframing, to emphasize disparate policing in primarily Black communities and widespread police brutality against the Black community. Indeed, in accordance with structuration theory (Giddens, 1984), agents have the power to make a difference to preexisting state of affairs. But agents also have to find some sense of security to effectively execute their responsibilities, and they achieve that level of security by routinizing and rationalizing relationships with significant others; this rationalization arises from practical consciousness, whereby agents have knowledge about what they do and the reasons for doing what they do. To be clear, such conditions may be favorable to effective counter-framing, which can transform preexisting state of affairs.

As per the Chauvin case, the judicial agents' counter-framing brought to light a new perspective because they functioned as a human agency, through making some difference to the preexisting state of affairs in matters of police violence against Blacks and other communities of color. Lest we forget, Black American history is overflowing with examples of how a stigmatized, racially disadvantaged, marginalized, and exploited group resisted the power of White slave owners, long before there were Civil Rights laws. And this happened because, notwithstanding their constant experiences of dehumanization and degradation, Blacks created choices and acted as a human agency. But the road traveled thus far is not enough to realize full racial equality and justice.

Racial domination sustains racial inequality and racism in all institutions. To substantially reduce or end racial inequality, including health inequalities, would necessitate a collective effort to dismantle racial domination. Giddens (1979) argues that the scope of people's discursive penetration within social systems of which they are participants is significant to the dialectic of control of collectivities, where there is a fundamental link between human agents and power. Giddens (1979, p. 6) further notes that

> power relations are always two-way; that is to say, however subordinate an actor may be in a social relationship, the very fact of involvement in that relationship gives him or her a certain amount of power over the other. Those in subordinate positions in social systems are frequently adept at converting whatever resources they possess into some degree of control over the conditions of reproduction of those social systems.

Feagin's work on the White racial frame (2020) is consistent with Giddens' finding on the power shared by subordinate actors or agents. Feagin posits that, at the individual level, subordinate groups could challenge the dominant White racial frame through "deframing," where an individual person can purposefully dissect a frame, to study all its features, and which may lead to some "reframing," to generate a new frame, so as to portray an issue differently. Bonilla-Silva's (2001) racialized social systems produce the ingredients for a racial hierarchy, generating superordinate (superior position) and subordinate (inferior or low-level position) social relations between the races. People at the top formulate views and practices supportive of the racial status quo, and people at the bottom assimilate views to challenge those positions articulated at the top level. Challenges by subordinate agents/communites of color are consistent with Giddens' dialectic of control (Giddens, 1979).

Any valid end to racial health disparities lies beyond the scope of the health system and health care. Structuration theory delivers power to the subordinate agents/communities of color through the duality of structure, which may be a potent pathway to actively consider toward dismantling systemic racism, the White racial frame, and the racialized social systems.

References

Abedi, V., Olulana, O., Avula, V., Chaudhary, D., Khan, A., Shahjouei, S., Li, J., & Zand, R. (2020). Racial, economic and health inequality and COVID-19 infection in the United States. *medRxiv*.

Alcendor, D. J. (2020). Racial disparities-associated COVID-19 mortality among minority populations in the US. *Journal of Clinical Medicine, 9*.

Anand, R., & Winters, M.-F. (2008). A retrospective view of corporate diversity training from 1964 to the present. *Academy of Management Learning & Education, 7*, 356–372.

Bailey, Z. D., Krieger, N., Agénor, M., Graves, J., Linos, N., & Bassett, M. T. (2017). Structural racism and health inequities in the USA: Evidence and interventions. *The Lancet, 389*, 1453–1463.

Bailey, Z. D., Feldman, J. M., & Bassett, M. T. (2021). *How structural racism works—Racist policies as a root cause of US racial health inequities*. Mass Medical Soc.

Bonilla-Silva, E. (1997). Rethinking racism: Toward a structural interpretation. *American Sociological Review*, 465–480.

Bonilla-Silva, E. (2001). *White supremacy and racism in the post-civil rights era*. Lynne Rienner Publishers.

Bonilla-Silva, E. (2013). *Racism without racists: Color-blind racism and the persistence of racial inequality in America*. Rowman & Littlefield Publishers.

Bonilla-Silva, E. (2015). More than prejudice: Restatement, reflections, and new directions in critical race theory. *Sociology of Race and Ethnicity, 1*, 73–87.

Bonilla-Silva, E. (2020). Color-blind racism in pandemic times. *Sociology of Race and Ethnicity*. https://doi.org/10.1177/2332649220941024

Boyd, R. W., Lindo, E. G., Weeks, L. D., & Mclemore, M. R. (2020). On racism: A new standard for publishing on racial health inequities. *Health Affairs Blog, 10*.

Byrd, W. M., & Clayton, L. A. (2012). *An American health dilemma: A medical history of African Americans and the problem of race: Beginnings to 1900*. Routledge.

Cabezas, C. (2021). Racism: A moral or explanatory concept? *Ethical Theory and Moral Practice*, 1–9.

Castle, B., Wendel, M., Kerr, J., Brooms, D., & Rollins, A. (2019). Public Health's approach to systemic racism: A systematic literature review. *Journal of Racial and Ethnic Health Disparities, 6*, 27–36.

CDC. (2021). *Provisional COVID-19 death counts by county and race* [online]. CDC. Available: https://data.cdc.gov/NCHS/Provisional-COVID-19-Death-Counts-by-County-and-Ra/k8wy-p9cg/data. Accessed 14 Apr 2021.

Collins, P. H., & Bilge, S. (2020). *Intersectionality*. Wiley.

Crenshaw, K. (1989). Demarginalizing the intersection of race and sex: A black feminist critique of antidiscrimination doctrine, feminist theory and antiracist politics. *u. Chi. Legal f.*, 139.

Cullen, P., Mackean, T., Worner, F., Wellington, C., Longbottom, H., Coombes, J., Bennett-Brook, K., Clapham, K., Ivers, R., Hackett, M., & Longbottom, M. (2020). *Trauma and Violence Informed Care Through Decolonising Interagency Partnerships: A Complexity Case Study of Waminda's Model of Systemic Decolonisation, International Journal of Environmental Research and Public Health*, 17.

Du Bois, W. E. B. (2007). *The Philadelphia negro*. Cosimo, Inc..

Feagin, J. R. (2001). Social justice and sociology: Agendas for the twenty-first century. *American Sociological Review, 66*.

Feagin, J. R. (2020). *The white racial frame: Centuries of racial framing and counter-framing*. Routledge.

Feagin, J., & Bennefield, Z. (2014). Systemic racism and US health care. *Social Science & Medicine, 103*, 7–14.

Ferber, A. L. (1998). Constructing whiteness: The intersections of race and gender in US white supremacist discourse. *Ethnic and Racial Studies, 21*, 48–63.

Frankenburg, R. (1993). *White women, race matters: The social construction of whiteness.* Routledge.

Gee, G. C., & Ford, C. L. (2011). Structural racism and health inequities: Old issues, new directions. *Du Bois Review: Social Science Research on Race, 8*, 115–132.

Geiger, H. J. (1996). *Race and health care—An American dilemma?* Mass Medical Soc.

Giddens, A. (1979). *Central problems in social theory: Action, structure, and contradiction in social analysis.* Univ of California Press.

Giddens, A. (1984). *The constitution of society: Outline of the theory of structuration.* Univ of California Press.

Golash-Boza, T. (2016). A critical and comprehensive sociological theory of race and racism. *Sociology of Race and Ethnicity, 2*, 129–141.

Gross, C. P., Essien, U. R., Pasha, S., Gross, J. R., Wang, S. Y., & Nunez-Smith, M. (2020). Racial and ethnic disparities in population-level Covid-19 mortality. *Journal of General Internal Medicine, 35*, 3097–3099.

Gu, T., Mack, J. A., Salvatore, M., Prabhu Sankar, S., Valley, T. S., Singh, K., Nallamothu, B. K., Kheterpal, S., Lisabeth, L., Fritsche, L. G., & Mukherjee, B. (2020). Characteristics associated with racial/ethnic disparities in COVID-19 outcomes in an academic health care system. *JAMA Network Open, 3*, e2025197.

Guess, T. J. (2006). The social construction of whiteness: Racism by intent, racism by consequence. *Critical Sociology, 32*, 649–673.

Hacker, A. (2010). *Two nations: Black and White, separate, hostile, unequal.* Simon and Schuster.

Hardeman, R. R. (2020). Examining racism in health services research: A disciplinary self-critique. *Health Services Research, 55*, 777.

Hardeman, R. R., Medina, E. M., & Kozhimannil, K. B. (2016). Structural racism and supporting black lives—The role of health professionals. *New England Journal of Medicine, 375*, 2113–2115.

Hardeman, R. R., Murphy, K. A., Karbeah, J. M., & Kozhimannil, K. B. (2018). Naming institutionalized racism in the public health literature: A systematic literature review. *Public Health Reports, 133*, 240–249.

Holtgrave, D. R., Barranco, M. A., Tesoriero, J. M., Blog, D. S., & Rosenberg, E. S. (2020). Assessing racial and ethnic disparities using a COVID-19 outcomes continuum for New York State. *Annals of Epidemiology, 48*, 9–14.

House, J. S., Kessler, R. C., & Herzog, A. R. (1990). Age, socioeconomic status, and health. *The Milbank Quarterly, 68*, 383–411.

Ignatiev, N., & Garvey, J. (1996). *Race traitor.* Psychology Press.

Jongen, C., Mccalman, J., Bainbridge, R., & Clifford, A. (2018). *Cultural competence in health: A review of the evidence.* Springer.

Kim, S. J., & Bostwick, W. (2020). Social vulnerability and racial inequality in COVID-19 deaths in Chicago. *Health Education & Behavior, 47*, 509–513.

King, G. (1996). Institutional racism and the medical/health complex: A conceptual analysis. *Ethnicity & Disease, 6*, 30–46.

Kinnamon, K., & Fabre, M. (Eds.). (1993). *Conversations with Richard Wright.* University Press of Mississippi.

Kopel, J., Perisetti, A., Roghani, A., Aziz, M., Gajendran, M., & Goyal, H. (2020). Racial and gender-based differences in COVID-19. *Frontiers in Public Health, 8*, 418.

Kullar, R., Marcelin, J. R., Swartz, T. H., Piggott, D. A., Macias Gil, R., Mathew, T. A., & Tan, T. (2020). Racial disparity of coronavirus disease 2019 in African American communities. *The Journal of Infectious Diseases, 222*, 890–893.

Laster Pirtle, W. N., & Wright, T. (2021). Structural gendered racism revealed in pandemic times: Intersectional approaches to understanding race and gender health inequities in COVID-19. *Gender & Society, 08912432211001302.*

Lavizzo-Mourey, R. J., Besser, R. E., & Williams, D. R. (2021). Understanding and mitigating health inequities—Past, current, and future directions. *New England Journal of Medicine, 384*, 1681–1684.

Li, D., Gaynor, S. M., Quick, C., Chen, J. T., Stephenson, B. J. K., Coull, B. A., & Lin, X. (2020). Unraveling US national COVID-19 racial/ethnic disparities using county level data among 328 million Americans. *medRxiv*.

Lieberson, S. (1987). *Making it count: The improvement of social research and theory*. Univ of California Press.

Link, B. G., & Phelan, J. (1995). Social conditions as fundamental causes of disease. *Journal of Health and Social Behavior*, 80–94.

Moore, J. T., Ricaldi, J. N., Rose, C. E., Fuld, J., Parise, M., Kang, G. J., Driscoll, A. K., Norris, T., Wilson, N., Rainisch, G., Valverde, E., Beresovsky, V., Agnew Brune, C., Oussayef, N. L., Rose, D. A., Adams, L. E., Awel, S., Villanueva, J., Meaney-Delman, D., & Honein, M. A. (2020). Disparities in Incidence of COVID-19 Among Underrepresented Racial/Ethnic Groups in Counties Identified as Hotspots During June 5–18, 2020–22 States, February–June 2020. *MMWR. Morbidity and Mortality Weekly Report, 69*, 1122–1126.

Myrdal, G. (1962). *An american dilemma*. Springer.

Nelson, A. (2002). Unequal treatment: Confronting racial and ethnic disparities in health care. *Journal of the National Medical Association, 94*, 666.

Nelson, H. D., Cantor, A., Wagner, J., Jungbauer, R., Quiñones, A., Stillman, L., & Kondo, K. (2020). Achieving health equity in preventive services: A systematic review for a national institutes of health pathways to prevention workshop. *Annals of Internal Medicine, 172*, 258–271.

Nummi, J., Jennings, C., & Feagin, J. (2019). *BlackLivesMatter: Innovative Black Resistance* (Wiley Online Library) (pp. 1042–1064). Sociological Forum.

Omi, M. & Winant, H. (1986). *Racial formation in the United States: from the 1960s to the 1980s*. Routledge & Kegan Paul.

Paradies, Y., Ben, J., Denson, N., Elias, A., Priest, N., Pieterse, A., Gupta, A., Kelaher, M., & Gee, G. (2015). Racism as a determinant of health: A systematic review and meta-analysis. *PLoS One, 10*, e0138511.

Phelan, J. C., & Link, B. G. (2015). Is racism a fundamental cause of inequalities in health? *Annual Review of Sociology, 41*, 311–330.

Raine, S., Liu, A., Mintz, J., Wahood, W., Huntley, K., & Haffizulla, F. (2020). Racial and ethnic disparities in COVID-19 outcomes: Social determination of health. *International Journal of Environmental Research and Public Health, 17*.

Reed, D. D. (2021). Racial disparities in healthcare: How COVID-19 ravaged one of the wealthiest African American counties in the United States. *Social Work in Public Health, 36*, 118–127.

Ritzer, G. (2011). *Sociological theory* (8th ed.). The McGrow Hill Companies.

Roberts, D. (2012). Debating the cause of health disparities implications for bioethics and racial equality. *Cambridge Q. Healthcare Ethics, 21*, 332.

Roediger, D. R. (1999). *The wages of whiteness: Race and the making of the American working class*. Verso.

Rogers, T. N., Rogers, C. R., Vansant-Webb, E., Gu, L. Y., Yan, B., & Qeadan, F. (2020). *Racial disparities in COVID-19 mortality among essential Workers in the United States*. World Med Health Policy.

Shepherd, S. M. (2019). Cultural awareness workshops: Limitations and practical consequences. *BMC Medical Education, 19*, 14.

Snowden, F. M. (2019). *Epidemics and society: From the black death to the present*. Yale University Press.

Tartof, S. Y., Qian, L., Hong, V., Wei, R., Nadjafi, R. F., Fischer, H., Li, Z., Shaw, S. F., Caparosa, S. L., Nau, C. L., Saxena, T., Rieg, G. K., Ackerson, B. K., Sharp, A. L., Skarbinski, J., Naik, T. K., & Murali, S. B. (2020). Obesity and mortality among patients diagnosed with

COVID-19: Results from an integrated health care organization. *Annals of Internal Medicine, 173*, 773–781.

The Sociologist. 2020. *Oppressive societies and social justice warriors: Conversation with Joe R. Feagin* [Online]. DCSS. Available: http://thesociologistdc.com/all-issues/oppressive-societies-and-social-justice-warriors-conversation-with-joe-r-feagin/. Accessed 5 June 2021.

Urquidez, A. G. (2020). *(Re-) defining racism: A philosophical analysis*. Springer.

Vahidy, F. S., Nicolas, J. C., Meeks, J. R., Khan, O., Pan, A., Jones, S. L., Masud, F., Sostman, H. D., Phillips, R., Andrieni, J. D., Kash, B. A., & Nasir, K. (2020). Racial and ethnic disparities in SARS-CoV-2 pandemic: Analysis of a COVID-19 observational registry for a diverse US metropolitan population. *BMJ Open, 10*, e039849.

Watson, S. D. (1994). Minority access and health reform: A civil right to health care. *The Journal of Law, Medicine & Ethics, 22*, 127–137.

West, C. (1994). *Race matters*. Vintage/Random House.

West, C. (2002). *Prophesy deliverance!: An afro-american revolutionary christianity*. Westminster John Knox Press.

Williams, D. R., & Mohammed, S. A. (2009). Discrimination and racial disparities in health: Evidence and needed research. *Journal of Behavioral Medicine, 32*, 20–47.

Williams, D. R., & Mohammed, S. A. (2013). Racism and health II: A needed research agenda for effective interventions. *American Behavioral Scientist, 57*, 1200–1226.

Witte, M. D. & Driscoll, S. (2021). *Chauvin guilty verdict is important, but more work needs to be done to advance racial justice, Stanford scholars say* [Online]. Stanford News, Stanford University. Available: https://news.stanford.edu/2021/04/20/what-the-verdict-means/. Accessed 8 June 2021.

Index